This Too Shall Pass

THIS TOO
SHALL PASS

BEING A CAREGIVER
FOR THE ELDERLY

Ginny Sisk

BROADMAN PRESS
NASHVILLE, TENNESSEE

© Copyright 1992 ● Broadman Press

All rights reserved

4260-26

ISBN: 0-8054-6026-8

Dewey Decimal Classification: 306.8

Subject Heading: FAMILY // ELDERLY - HOME CARE

Library of Congress Card Catalog Number: 91-1194

Printed in the United States of America

Unless otherwise stated, Scripture quotations are from the *King James Version.*

Scripture quotations marked TLB are from *The Living Bible.* Copyright © Tyndale House Publishers, Wheaton, Illinois, 1971. Used by permission.

Scripture quotations marked NIV are from the Holy Bible, *New International Version,* copyright © 1973, 1978, 1984 by International Bible Society.

Sisk, Ginny, 1927-

    This too shall pass / Ginny Sisk.

      p.   cm.

    Includes bibliographical reference.

    ISBN 0-8054-6026-8

    1. Aging parents--Care--United States. 2. Aging parents--Health and hygiene--United States. 3.Adult children--United States--Psychology. 4. Old age--United States. 5. Cancer--Patients--Family relationships. 6. Alzheimer's disease--Patients--Family relationships. I. Title.

HV1461.S55 1991

362.1'96831--dc20   91-1194

                                                       CIP

Dedicated to Ted Sisk, the one who has encouraged and pushed me to live to my full potential, who has allowed me to be my own person; who invited me to be his partner in ministry, his confidante, his critic, his lover, the mother of his four wonderful sons and, most importantly, his wife.

To the glory of Christ, I also dedicate this work, praying it will bless and lighten the load of some worn caregiver.

Acknowledgments

My thanks to all those who have "picked up the slack" in my responsibilities. I am grateful to my sons, Larry, Jon, Paul, and Mark, who reassured me, helped me with recall, editing, and suggestions. A special thanks to Paul and my husband, Ted, for teaching me to use the word processor and for their hours of correcting and editing.

I am deeply indebted to Kathy Gannoe, the Bluegrass Long-term Care Ombudsman for my area, who made her library and research files accessible to me. Perusing through these files gave me an invaluable educational opportunity.

My friends who were willing to give me an interview and relate their stories, did so with much pain and emotion as they remembered. Sometimes it was a personal sacrifice in time and energy to share. Some are still in the throes of these experiences. These personal things are told that you might be encouraged to hang in there.

To those who shared their stories but wish to remain anonymous, I am grateful.

Contents

Introduction

Ten years ago if someone had suggested to me that I would one day be contemplating writing a book of any kind, much less one on the care of the elderly, I would have dismissed the idea. After all, we didn't really have elderly parents, just wonderful mature ones who could take care of themselves.

That scenario soon changed, however, when our family went through the throes of cancer and Alzheimer's disease. We literally turned our house into a hospice.

Before this story began, I felt I was the most blessed woman in all the world. I had a wonderful pastor-husband who loved me totally and exclusively and who shared his ministry with me. I had four handsome, healthy sons, and later five delightful, beautiful grandchildren. I had always been the beloved daughter-in-law who enjoyed member-of-the-family status. My world was on a string, and I was pulling it along. It seemed too good to be true.

The main characters in this book are Theodore Roosevelt Sisk, Sr., and Lena Smith Sisk, his wife of fifty years who had borne his two children, Theodore Roosevelt Sisk, Jr., (Ted) and Ruth Sisk Pleak. Jesse Lovell Sisk and Etta Williams Sisk were the paternal grandparents who lived in the big old house on West Doyle Street in Toccoa, Georgia.

Theodore and Lena Sisk had really moved in with Grandpa and Granny Sisk on their wedding night after having eloped and with nowhere else to go. Grandpa informed Theodore that if he was man enough to take a wife, he was man enough to support her and take care of her. But it was a cold December night in 1926 and as they walked down the street to they-did-not-know-where, Grandpa ran after them crying and saying, "Come on back, I didn't mean what I said!" And so the two families merged into one for the rest of the elder Sisks's lives. Ted and Ruth grew up with two sets of parents, or so it seemed to them.

Nothing but love was shown me as I became a part of the Sisk family. Because my own mother had died when I was fourteen, Lena, who had been my mother's friend, became my mother in a very real sense. She was always there when our children came along: and later, when we needed to make a trip, she and Theodore came to keep the boys. This was fairly easy since Theodore was self-employed most of that time. My children feel they had the greatest grandparents in the world. Just recently, our second son, Jon, remarked to us that he fondly remembers his grandfather's unabashed glee when welcoming him as a kid. The Sisks and I didn't always agree on everything, but we always knew we disagreed in love with no hard feelings.

If I were to write an epitaph for my father-in-law, I would have to say that he drank deeply from the cup of life. He was a handsome, gifted musician who knew how to make people feel good about themselves. He was generous to a fault, mischievous yet peaceful, a lover of people, especially his family. He was a Christian but not a religious fanatic, a consoler, one who never met a stranger, and so affable that others felt at ease around him.

Years ago, when Theodore started smoking, no one knew of the health hazards involved as we do today. It was he who gave my boys their first cigarettes. I wish he hadn't, but I know he would never knowingly have done anything that he felt would harm them. Later, he was to realize how fatal smoking can be. Even after his surgery, equipped with a prosthesis with which he could not smoke, he would slip a cigarette and put it in his mouth and inhale trying to get some smell of tobacco sensation. He was still addicted to nicotine.

My mother-in-law was like the Rock of Gibraltar that could not be shaken in her faith and devotion to her family and her Lord. A modest, patient woman who held her head high and shared her hospitality with all who came her way, expected or unexpected. She was frugal, yet practical and generous. She was as faithful to her church as she could be considering their life-style of always being gone to some other church for a singing school, revival, or singing convention.

Who knows how long Alzheimer's disease was been around? We used to call it everything from old age to senility. Even when we realized that something terrible was wrong with Lena, more than ten years before she died, we attributed it to hardening of the arteries—supposedly from high blood pressure. Much of that was chalked up to eating too many fried foods and the lack of other nutritional knowledge. We still don't know what causes Alzheimer's disease, how people contract it or develop it, and surely not the cure. In my opinion, it is the most degrading, humiliating disease one can have, because it robs the individual of his dignity and personality and eventually his independence and reasoning power.

I am writing this book not to tell our family story per se but to share with others how we coped (or were unable to cope) with this horrible intrusion in our lives. Hopefully, it will give courage and inspiration to those who are going through this same trauma. I pray it will give some insight for others who may have to deal with caring for the sick and elderly.

My personal faith in God and the solid support of my husband and church family made my load a lot easier to carry than it would have been for those who have no support system or supernatural strength from which to draw.

In parts I and II I have tried to tell our story and how we managed. You will find that part III has a different character. It is written to give you the benefit of research, both mine and that of some experts. It does not purport to be a comprehensive work.

Part III is intended to give you information and insight about the diseases and afflictions of old age. It is hoped that any misconceptions you have about old age, illness, or caregiving responsibilities will be cleared up. No book or literary piece will have all the answers. This section doesn't pretend to replace medical advice and help. It is not all inclusive. Every family situation is different and each person who is the primary caregiver has his or her own story to tell.

I can identify with the pain other families experience because I remember so well that at times I appeared to be dragging my feet in writing it. I know now that I was subconsciously dreading the pain of going back and reliving some of those emotions.

Part I:

Light at the End of the Tunnel

1

"In the Beginning . . ."

"Ted, come in here!" an emotion-filled voice called to us as we stood in the cold, dimly lit, long white corridor on the third floor of the hospital, in the very early hours of this September morning. We were awaiting the exit of the nurse who had gone in to give Dad his pre-op shot in preparation for his surgery that was scheduled for this morning on which fog fell like a gray shroud across Augusta, Georgia.

The nurse appeared in the doorway of Dad's semiprivate room, looking as bewildered as we were, only with a hint of impatience. Dad's voice had surely awakened the sleeping patient in the other bed. At this very last minute Dad was about to refuse to have the radical facial surgery for cancer that might prolong his life a few more months. Ted quickly entered the room, and as Mama and I stood waiting outside we could hear voices but could not really understand what was being said. Suddenly we heard Dad's high-pitched, frightened voice as he said to Ted and the nurse waiting with a needle in her hand, "I'm not sure that I want to go through with this! Maybe I'll just go on and die now and get it over with! Then, you won't have to be bothered with me anymore!"

It was obvious from this last expression of apprehension that he was remembering we had driven down from Kentucky, taking a week of vacation, to be with him during this ordeal: surgically removing a fast growing, cancerous tumor that had invaded his sinus cavities, nose, mouth, and perhaps even now would mean the loss of at least one eye. Earlier Dad had mentioned repeatedly that

16

he was sorry he was putting us to so much trouble and causing us to use our vacation time like this. No amount of reassurance could convince him that we had wanted to be here with him, to stand by him, to lend support to Mama (who was almost as frightened as he was), and to love and pray for him.

Calmly, but emphatically, Ted reminded him of the terrible pain he had been suffering these last eight or nine months as he had undergone the attempted "cures" inflicted upon him by a number of doctors who were treating him for severe sinusitis.

During the summer which had just passed, when they had spent some days in Kentucky and he had suffered so much, Ted had given his father an ultimatum. Either he give his word that he would seek specialized medical help when he returned to Georgia or we would keep him in Lexington to see that he got it. Dad had promised he would. He kept his word, seeing doctors at the University of Georgia Medical Center at Augusta. The diagnosis was almost more than we could bear; and yet, we were not really surprised. Though he had celebrated his seventy-first birthday in July the doctors encouraged him to go ahead with the surgery describing to him in detail what was probably involved and how they felt they could help him.

Finally, now as he sat on the edge of his hospital bed smoking the last cigarette he would ever smoke, he nodded to the nurse with the long, sedative-filled needle, to go ahead. He slowly turned on his side, raised the hospital jacket from his hip, and took the shot that was to begin this ordeal.

As the nurse left the room and hurried down the long corridor, Mama and I edged back toward the door and saw this dear face filled with resignation and the very evident feeling that he had thrust himself upon the mercy and grace of his Heavenly Father. As Ted stood by his bed, stroking his dad's hand, we all knew that God's grace would indeed be sufficient for all of us in the days to follow. At that moment, none of us realized how deeply we would be drawing from this well of mercy and grace.

After the prescribed time, the surgical team came for him and he climbed on the gurney unassisted. We watched from the hall as they rolled him by and Mama bent down to kiss him. I was glad that we had already prayed together before he became groggy.

Ted and I returned to his room briefly. I watched as Ted walked over to the cabinet by the bed that houses the bedpan, soap dish, wash pan, and other incidentals, and saw him open the drawer to see what was inside. There was a little change, a few family pictures, and a half pack of cigarettes and a lighter. Ted took the cigarettes and the lighter. At this point, I was reminded of having heard Dad say many times, "I have helped make tobacco companies rich while they have made me a pauper and their cigarettes have killed me with cancer!"

The three of us slowly made our way to the surgical waiting room to begin the long, quiet vigil that would last into the afternoon while Dad was in surgery. We tried to make small talk at first and I made some effort to be a bit lighthearted, but it was superficial and meaningless for all of us. Longer and longer periods of silence began to fall over us. Finally, Ted got up to walk around, maybe to be alone; I was sure he was remembering the better, happier days of his growing up with one of the best dads ever. No, he was not a perfect example, but no one could ever doubt that Theodore Sisk loved his family, especially his children, and was so proud of their accomplishments. He loved Paul Pleak, his son-in-law, and me as his own. He loved children and, I think, would have loved to have had more than just Ted and Ruth. His grandchildren were a real joy to him, and they loved him dearly. My boys especially loved the tales he would tell and the faces he would make.

The drive down from Kentucky to Georgia is usually one of anticipation and delight as we pass through the mountains of Kentucky and Tennessee, then finally into the flat lands of Middle and South Georgia, where Mama and Dad have made their home the last few years. Dad directed the music in the Alexander Baptist

Church. This trip had been different. We were quieter, almost like waiting for a jury to return with an expected verdict of guilty. For days we had been fearful of how serious Dad's condition really was.

2

"Ah, How Sweet It Was"

In the quietness of the waiting, my mind began to wonder, too. Dad loved to tell that he once courted my mother, Woody Garrison Dalton, before my dad married her. It must not have been too serious because our families have remained friends through the years. It was a natural thing, since Ted's dad and my father had been good friends from the time my dad stayed in the Sisk home in Toccoa, Georgia, while he attended a state Sunday School rally back in the 1920s. The friendship lasted through the years as our families visited from time to time.

I remembered the times when we were children and the families visited back and forth. There was never enough bed space, so the kids slept on the floor on pallets made of the many handmade quilts that were in each of our homes. Once, when Ted, Ruth, and I had been put to bed on the floor and Ted kept reaching over Ruth to touch me, Ruth screamed her head off to make sure her mother knew what "Junior" was doing.

It was an easy thing for me to fall in love with handsome Ted Sisk when I was sixteen. Though many objected to our getting married at nineteen, I don't recall that Theodore Sisk ever voiced one word of objection. Rather, he seemed pleased. From the time I came into the Sisk family, I was treated like a daughter, and I loved him like my own father. He was always encouraging and affirming me, especially about my cooking and homemaking. He loved to eat. It was no wonder he loved my cooking—Ted's mother had taught me much of what I know about cooking and sewing.

I remembered once when we lived in Banks County, Georgia, that he came by unexpectedly one Saturday night and we were just about to sit down to a simple dinner of sausage, grits, eggs, hot biscuits, and sorghum. At our invitation he joined us. He ate heartily and then said, "I wish Lena would ever fix something like that!" She did, almost every morning for breakfast.

I thought of the piano students he had had, of all the songs he has written, many of which are still being sung today by major gospel groups. A familiar picture is one of Dad with a manuscript pad and pencil sitting at the piano writing and singing his newest creation often without words, just do-re-mi's. Hearing him call to Mama in the kitchen, "Lena, come here and sing this tune with me!" meant that took precedence over whatever she was doing at the time. For as long as Ted can remember, his dad had written music and had taught his children to read music—even before they could read the words to songs. He now had "grandchildren" in gospel music, not biological grandchildren but "music grandchildren." I thought of the times when we were courting and had gone with the family on a weekend singing engagement instead of the traditional date, of the stolen moments when Ted and I would sneak out of the church and back to the car to have a few minutes alone. Later that afternoon or evening we would drive back home so everyone could be there for school or work the next day. Dad never had a great deal of interest in many things other than his music and things related to it. Oh, I didn't mean to leave out his love for checkers. I smiled a little to myself as I remembered how fervently he and Ted would play and the verbal banter that took place between them. Still he was a poor sport when Ted beat him at his own game. I understand he had won some state championships years before.

The night our first child, Larry, was born I wanted to throw both Ted and his dad out for staying up half the night playing checkers. I could not go to sleep for their constant meaningless chatter and I was so weary and big (also a little exasperated because I had already been to the hospital on a false alarm eight days earlier). Since we lived out in the country on the church field of our first pastorate, we stayed in Toccoa to be close to the Stephens County Hospital and each night Ted and Dad played checkers to pass the time. I paid them back though, because just about time they all got to sleep, Larry decided it was time for him to make his debut and we woke up the whole house.

I remembered how Dad could hardly wait to hold his first grandchild. He and Mama were always so available to come to keep our kids when we went to conventions and other church meetings. I owe my daughters-in-law a lot of baby-sitting, for I have surely had a lot of help from my in-laws.

My troubled mind now preferred to continue to think of happier days—especially when we were first married and had our first country pastorate. When there was a free evening, we would drive from Banks County to Toccoa, uninvited and unannounced, to have dinner with the entire Sisk family— Grandpa, Granny, Mama, and Dad. It was not unusual to make homemade ice cream in a crank freezer, cook hamburgers on the grill or fry chicken or steak, and make hot biscuits and gravy. The men would play checkers while we washed dishes and talked. I think I never felt more family love than I did during those early days of our marriage and family. There was never a time when I didn't feel I was a welcomed part of the Sisk family.

My family, the Daltons, rarely visited us after we left our first pastorate at Harmony Baptist Church, Baldwin, Georgia, to go to The Southern Baptist Theological Seminary in Louisville, Kentucky. Later, we went to the First Baptist Church, Hogansville, Georgia. However, the Sisks visited frequently wherever we lived. Every time we had a new baby, Mrs. Sisk was there to mother me and the rest of the family. I could hardly believe that now we had come to this state of trauma in all our lives.

I recalled with delight and amusement the many funny stories that Dad always seemed to have. Some would bear repeating-- some would not. He enjoyed life to the fullest. He had never made a lot of money and had saved practically none but he had taught his children how to love and to enjoy life and people. He had taught me a lot of things, too, that I shall always treasure. He was without a doubt one of the most colorful characters I've ever known. Could this now be the beginning of the end? I felt a new kind of fear, and I didn't like it.

For the thousandth time we went over again why this cancer should strike Dad in the facial area. Surely, we knew it was the effect of smoking, but we had never heard of anyone having cancer of the sinuses. We asked Mama if any other family members had had any apparent weakness in this area. But asking her was folly because of the Alzheimer's disease; she could not even remember family members' names or where they lived—not even when we tried to help her by telling her what we recalled. Then, we, grasping as if for the proverbial straw began to say, "Well, maybe if he had done this or that," but really having no basis for those remarks.

I preferred to think of those wonderful days when we gathered with all the family at Toccoa for Christmas or Thanksgiving, or even for birthdays to hear again tales of the past or plans for the future. It might be to listen to the strains of a new song Dad was writing, or in the summertime sit on the cool front porch that wrapped itself halfway around the house in the large, many-times-painted rockers as we strung beans or shelled peas. Often, Granny Sisk darned socks with a light bulb run into the toe or heel. Sometimes I would just sit, rock, and thumb through women's magazines I couldn't afford to subscribe to at the time. Often neighbors would come by and stop and chat for a few minutes as we exchanged news of the community.

I was abruptly brought back to the present as Ted was finally summoned by a nurse to go to a designated phone to talk to the doctors from the operating suite. I rushed with Ted to the phone and pressed my ear against his head so I could hear, too. My heart was racing as I waited for the verdict. *Would he lose his eye? Did they get it all?* The surgery was completed and Dad was in recovery. They had been able to confine it to the face, palate, and sinuses, though, there seemed to be a questionable spot on his lung. He did *not* lose his eye. I breathed a prayer of thanksgiving. Again, I thought how gracious is our Heavenly Father! There would be no chemotherapy—only radiation therapy. This seemed strange to us considering the seriousness of the surgery, but we surely didn't question the doctors about it. We knew that chemotherapy often makes patients extremely nauseated, and obviously Dad couldn't cope with that without running the risk of choking.

3

The Grim Reality of a Changing Life-style

The days of recuperation were long and tedious. This once-debonair, good-looking man who attracted the attention of all the women and girls by his uninhibited, friendly way, as well as his handsome face and his beautiful voice, was now faced with this grotesque hole in his face as large as a small grapefruit. He would have to learn to use a special prosthesis that would be made to cover this cavern; it would include his dentures, his palate, his nose, and whatever else was necessary to give him some semblance of his former self.

Later that year, Dr. Barry M. Goldman, Director of the University of Georgia's Maxillofacial Services Division said in an article in *The Atlanta Constitution*, "It is the most psychologically devastating surgery. Our job is to rehabilitate those patients."[1] In the article, he was speaking of the kind of surgery Dad had received and of the prosthesis that was being constructed. Rehabilitation included the construction of what looked like part of a mask that was glued to the patient's face.

Dad's reluctance to have the surgery was understandable. Doubtless, he had weighed the well-known and often-experienced pain with the now deformed face that looked back at him from the mirror like a stranger. His upper lip and palate were gone! Only from the eyes up and the lower lip down could he have recognized himself. How could he possibly face his friends and colleagues in this condition? Thank God for the bandages that covered his face, at least for the moment. We all had our turn at nausea when we looked at his face.

Fortunately, when he first viewed himself in the bathroom mirror at the hospital, he did not understand or know of the long, discouraging hours and days that lay ahead as he had to learn to use this specially built prosthesis, the first of its kind to be made for this particular type of facial surgery. At the insistence of his doctors, however, he quickly learned to use his prosthesis. That in itself involved patience as he worked with the many parts that made up the prosthesis. The tape, the glue, and the horror of seeing oneself in the mirror, made his hands shake almost uncontrollably. No wonder he wept.

He strongly resented the medical students who came in to watch. The Medical Center at Augusta is a teaching hospital for the University of Georgia. Dad often felt they were just curious, not really realizing that perhaps by watching his progress, they might be able someday to do for another what had been done for him. He was especially resentful when they gathered just outside his door to evaluate and critique his progress. Later, he would boast, however, that he was the first to use this prosthesis and proudly he would show the newspaper article describing its use and noting its developer.

So often the Lord has someone in the wings to give that added spiritual dimension to a situation—this was no different. One of the staff physicians was so kind to take the time to explain in detail and in layman's terminology just what would be taking place during the surgery. The physician talked not only about the medical aspect of this situation but also about the spiritual. He assured Dad that he personally would be praying for him. This was reassuring to all of us.

Another helpful new friend was Dad's roommate, a man from Middle Georgia who was facing the prospects of losing his leg because of severe diabetes. For some reason, Dad did not go into intensive care immediately following surgery and this man would ring for the nurses or attendants to care for Dad since he could not due to the tracheotomy. We were glad this dear man was occupying the other bed. For brief periods when we were away, his wife was caring for both patients.

4

How Long Can They Hold On?

The day finally came when Dad could leave the hospital and return to their home next door to the church where he had been serving. With only a bandage covering the monstrous hole in his face, he walked out of the hospital with his head high belying the fear, hurt, and perhaps even embarrassment he felt.

Driving into the small community in the deep South where he was known and loved by all, he expressed a measure of cautious gratitude to God and to his friends for all they had done for him.

He loved the little house with three rooms down each side and the front porch and stoop which sheltered the front door from the rain. The white siding needed a coat of paint and the scraggly yard needed to be cleared of the twigs and limbs which had been blown off by a recent wind, but that could wait. Yet, it was home—not like the stately old house he had left in Toccoa but it was really all they could care for. It had provided adequately for the two of them and for family and friends as they had visited, so it satisfied him.

He had waved at the whittlers, tobacco chewers, and "government runners" sitting on the benches and nail kegs as he had passed the country store just before they crossed the railroad and drove up by the church and into his own yard.

But with all his courage displayed to the public, he was scared.

In a few weeks he was driving again with his glasses held over his eyes with pieces of cellophane tape (because he had no nose for the glasses to rest on at that time).

We could not stay in Georgia long enough to see him home

from the hospital and Ruth, Ted's sister, was not nearby either. They were quite dependent on the church community to get Mama back and forth to the hospital. These days of recuperation were more difficult for Ruth since she lived closer than we did. The trips to Augusta while Dad was hospitalized and later to Alexander were nerve-racking and draining. We, in Lexington, felt pulled and drawn to share in this responsibility but bound by distance and our obligations to Immanuel Baptist Church and our own family, were locked out. We often found ourselves joining Ruth in her prayer, "Lord, whatever You are trying to teach us, please help us learn quickly!"

Dad was to live long enough to teach us many things. We learned, like the apostle Paul, that we must be content in whatever state we find ourselves.

Fifteen months later at the celebration of their fiftieth wedding anniversary, Dad played his part perfectly as he joined us in welcoming guests all afternoon. Mama looked beautiful in her long dress. She was a stately lady who carried herself erect. Her modesty was one of her virtues. Although life had not always been easy, her smiling face on this their special day gave no indication of that. Indeed, she was the grand dame of our family. Her granddaughters made up her face and did her hair. Many people who came to call really had no idea how sick either of them was at that time.

As we all gathered for the anniversary celebration, there was an ominous feeling among all of us that this might be the last time we'd gather at their home for any sort of celebration as we had been accustomed to doing. Of course, Ruth and I had made all the preparations for the anniversary party, which meant bringing food and serving things from Lexington and Marietta. It was a pleasure and we wanted to do this for them and for us.

Ted and I made a week of it as we took our family and went down right after Christmas to get things in order. We even entertained some old friends of theirs a few days before, and this seemed to please both of them.

The day of the party was beautiful and mild, not unusual in

Middle Georgia for winter. Many friends of years gone by came. It was a good day and we were all glad we had done it, but it wasn't easy. Getting the house ready for that kind of party took a lot of work because all around was evidence that Mama had lost her housekeeping skills. Worse still, she was unaware that she had. Fortunately, she was very congenial and whatever we wanted to do was fine with her. When it was over, they were both exhausted and we had mixed emotions—both joy and sadness, The celebration seemed to have a note of finality.

Months earlier Dad had reached the place where he could begin to pick up the pieces of his life again. He was able to sing again, and rather acceptably, in spite of the prosthesis. He still loved to show his expertise on the piano and perhaps imagined hearing his once lovely tenor voice as it had been before it was marred with sixty years of cigarette smoking and now with surgery. He attempted to resume his responsibilities as minister of music in the small country church. It was to this church they had come when they sold the old home place on Doyle Street in Toccoa.

His church responsibility was too much, physically and emotionally, and eventually he had to resign. He so wanted to continue his church work that he waited too long (or perhaps we let him wait too long) to resign. We, his family, had no idea how bad things really were with them until a committee from the church notified us that they felt Dad and Mama were not capable of taking care of themselves anymore. Adding to the embarrassment Dad felt was the realization that he just couldn't carry on as he previously had. He was hurt with the church people and felt betrayed, but they were right. We were embarrassed that we had let this situation exist so long, but when we would talk to Dad and Mama, or rather to him, he would give us the impression that all was going well. Admittedly, he would complain that he didn't know what he was going to do with Mama—she seemed to be losing her mind, he would say.

Dad's mood swings were just what one would expect them to be—up and down. He would have crying jags and would show his impatience with Mama at her lack of understanding and remembering, while the next minute he would realize that she couldn't help it and then he would hold her in his arms with the evident feeling that he didn't know how long he would have the privilege of holding her. They seemed to quarrel more and more often. Both were scared, each trying to cover for the other.

For as long as I can remember Mama would always feed him what she felt he should have, whether it was what he wanted or not. It became a family joke because she would always ask him if he wanted one egg or two, then proceed to fix him two, because he always said he wanted one. As long as she could, she continued to do that but it was no longer a joke with them but rather became a source of contention. Day by day it was becoming more and more evident to all of us that life would never be the same again—for them or for us, their children.

5

The Heartbreak of Unending Change

Next came the stark reality that we had to get Dad and Mama closer to us, and the sooner the better. It was a dismal day when we started the task of moving them; it was rainy and chilly. They had talked about the advisability of coming to Lexington to be near us. Or should they move to Marietta to be near Ruth? A number of things were in favor of moving to Marietta. For one thing, Georgia had always been their home. Another factor was being nearer the Georgia Medical Center in Augusta. Although they loved Lexington and our church people, they decided to go to Marietta. By now, the "insignificant" spot on his lung had become very suspicious.

Later Ruth was to question the wisdom of their being so close, since they immediately became so dependent upon her. Dad and Mama seemed to be quarreling more frequently and her mind was getting worse. It was dangerous to let Mama cook with a gas stove for fear she would brush her clothing too close to a burner or create some other hazard. Besides, she had forgotten how to cook.

Once she would have burned the apartment house down by leaving bacon drippings in the skillet and turning the unit to "high" instead of "off," had Dad not been there to put out the fire. They were eating more and more fast foods. This fear of what might happen next and of constant watching her by Dad was taking its toll. To say the situation was getting bad was a gross understatement. We were later to learn just how much he did for Mama and how much he covered for her in public, trying to make her appear normal. Only later did we determine that she was unable to do many things that we had assumed she could still do.

He was not getting stronger, rather he seemed to be going down-hill almost daily. It was turning out to be a day-by-day thing. How much longer could they live alone, even in Marietta?

They were like children tattling on each other to Ruth, whose nerves had about reached the breaking point. Dad would often go to the library where Ruth was librarian, to unload on her, much to her chagrin, with the library full of patrons. Obviously, he was caught between the realization of his own deteriorating condition, his helplessness at being unable to improve either his situation or Mama's, his fear and concern over what was happening to Mama, and the knowledge that he could do little to improve any of it. Ruth was nearby, so she became his sounding board. His exaspera-tion spilled over onto her.

Fortunately, Dad could still drive fairly safely and this allowed them to shop for a few prepared foods, go to the gas station, to the dry cleaners, and to the post office. Being able to go the post office to buy stamps and mail letters and cards has always been a big thing with Dad. He was undoubtedly the greatest correspondent I have ever known. He seemed to feel a real need as well as pleasure to frequently write his children, grandchildren, and his friends. Some of this compulsion was a carryover from the days of the Sisk Music Company when they had songbooks to mail to customers almost daily.

More often than not, they ate their evening meal with Ruth. At least that way she could see that they had a balanced diet and ate regularly. Besides it was easier than going over to their place to fix something.

The Alzheimer's disease caused Mama to take less and less in-terest in her apartment or to be concerned about food, laundry, housecleaning or even personal hygiene. This was such a depar-ture from her former way of life when she took so much pride in herself, her house, and in her cooking and sewing ability. I owe so much to her for teaching me things about keeping house, cooking, and so many things in general. She was indeed the mother I had lost as a teenage girl. One of the fun things we did was to swap recipes or try out new ones together.

Those days were lost forever now. In the earlier days of her illness when she was aware that something was wrong but she did not know what, she would ask, "Am I losing my mind?" and we would reassure her that she was not but that she had hardening of the arteries of the brain that caused her to forget.

6

The Long Road

They were worn out from the long trip, all four of them. It was
not helped by the bickering that went on in the car between Mama
and Dad on the long, nearly four-hundred-mile trip from Marietta
to Lexington. Frequent stops were necessary and that extended
the travel time. Finding the right place to eat was also a problem.
Dad didn't like to eat in public with his prosthesis which had to be
cleaned well afterwards. In a rest room, adults and children alike
would stare at him taking all that apparatus apart and cleaning it.
It added to his misery.

When they finally arrived at our house, all faces revealed the
weariness of the trip and the relief at being released from the close
confinement of the car. Dad was the last to come through the
kitchen door, and I was shaken by the ashen look on his face. We
had not seen him in several weeks. I had such an uneasy feeling,
but after embracing and greeting everyone he seemed to perk up a
little and we felt better. While we felt fairly safe about his driving
around Marietta, none of us had felt he should attempt the long
trip to Lexington, just the two of them, so Ruth and Paul had
dropped them by as they were on their way to Indiana to see Paul's
father. Ruth was so physically and emotionally tired that she appeared ill herself. Hopefully, a good night's sleep would make her
feel better. We never dreamed that this visit of Ted's parents to our
home would be their last together, or that it would extend through
his father's death.

The time was early December, and they had planned to stay

with us several weeks—perhaps even until spring. At that time we would drive them home or they would fly. Dad hated to fly, but the trip was so hard on him we were confident he would consent. The next morning, after a good rest, everyone seemed better. Once more we latched on to a tiny thread of hope and encouragement. Dad seemed to take pride in getting himself bathed, dressed, and the prosthesis in place so he could go out "looking decent." He looked forward to the church services on Sunday but was reluctant to go to the family-night dinners on Wednesday. He felt he had become somewhat of a messy eater and was afraid that people would stare, as indeed they often did. He became very embarrassed and irritated, even at children, when people stared. Most of the time, the prothesis was hardly noticeable since it was so nearly his natural skin tones.

At church everyone was exceedingly gracious and tried hard to make them feel comfortable. Many times when asked how he was, he would reply that he was great. Other times he would show his deep depression and fear by his replies.

For as long as I have known Theodore Sisk he has wanted to be top man on the totem pole. He wanted to draw attention to himself. Often, for example, when he was visiting us, he would go to the piano at the end of the postlude following worship and play and sing uninvited. But he had such a winsome way that it was no time at all until he would have a crowd around him encouraging him to play some more. For some strange reason, Dad felt that Ted upstaged him when Ted preached and all eyes were on him. Dad was torn between his pride in Ted and the need of his own self-aggrandizement. For some reason Dad needed to bathe his ego in the limelight.

I can remember times on other visits to Lexington when he would open cellophane-wrapped candy, talk, or write notes during prayer or preaching and seem to enjoy people turning to see who was doing it. This seemed to get worse as he grew more ill. Often I would reach across Mama gently to place my hand on his to quieten the paper rustling or unwrapping procedures. Never did he act as if he minded, but seemed more like a little boy caught. Another attention getter he had was "loving on Mama" in public, especially church. She would be embarrassed and would turn him a cold shoulder but he knew that would tickle all who saw him. He was a performer to the end. He loved center stage with all the lights and fanfare. He was a flatterer and a charmer; females of all ages ate that up—me included.

Music and singing for others were so much a part of the very fiber of his being that he seemed to hold on to that longer than any other activity—even checkers. He was often peeved because Ted could not stop his work and play checkers. Sometimes he would insist that Mama play with him. She was never a challenge for him and now she could not do anything right, so he would move both sides of the board or take her hand and move the right piece.

Our church friends knew how difficult it was for him and how the time dragged for him each day. A dear friend of ours who had an aged mother and dad, called to ask if Dad would like to come to her house on a given night to play and sing for her parents and an aunt. He was so excited he could hardly wait for the time to come for her to pick him up. For two hours, he played his own songs and sang for them, told tall tales for their amusement and had a ball. Mama had always been jealous of Dad (little wonder) and even at that age and that condition, she still was jealous of " Mis' Lib." She stood at the front door and fussed because he was so late—wondering what he could be doing. She couldn't remember where he had gone but felt he should be home with her. She couldn't express her jealousy but she was uncomfortable.

We tried to give them all the time we could, especially during this last visit, but their resentment grew because of our involvement with the church. We later found cruel, heartrending notes that Dad had written, almost as if they were addressed "To Whom It May Concern." These notes expressed his hurt with his family, his friends, and even his government. One such note we found was entitled "Something to Remember" and went like this.

"I eat too much, I write too much, these are things I have been asked to do. I had to give up cigarettes because I was fussed at so much by my wife and everybody else, and Dr. said so, too. Now I got nothing to help me calm down when the weak spells hit me, but that's OK. Operation Sept. 7th, 1976, Talmidge [sic] Hospital, Augusta, GA., Dr. Johnson, Dr. Jones, the best. Dentist Dr. Goldman, eye specialist Dr. Ramadon. Nine months ago today, June 7th, 1977, still no nose or teeth, I have been so discouraged."

We knew they were the thoughts of a very ill man who was terribly frightened. His mood swings were increasingly evident.

Though they had been with us for weeks now, they still somehow felt they were visiting and resented the little time that Ted had to give them. Dad wanted Ted to sing with him, take him for a ride, or listen to him relive some special episodes in his life. This was important to him and to us, and we were genuinely sorry for the lack of time we had to give, but that is part of being a pastor of a large metropolitan church.

Dad complained because he didn't have his car and that we never offered him ours to drive. We got the feeling sometimes that he did not believe us when we had to be away for meetings. If we had to be gone overnight, we asked Paul and Nancy Anderson, our next-door neighbors, to come over, but to Mama and Dad it was not the same. Our son Mark, who was twenty and living at home attending the University of Kentucky, was regarded by them as "just a kid." They considered themselves to be alone with just Mark there.

Mama tried to do things for Dad to be helpful but her own mental condition did not allow her to think clearly, so rather than help, she would do foolish things that annoyed him. Before he got too ill to eat at the table, Mama would put food on his plate that she thought he should have even though he told her he did not want it. She still did that—much to his consternation and annoyance.

He was worried over his own physical condition and her mental condition. The stress of his illness was making her condition worse, too. Her various and sundry emotions tore at her. At one time, she would be filled with gratitude to me for the things I did for Dad and at other times jealous of those things that she knew she should be able to do for him and couldn't. Once when I helped him with the urinal after he became bedridden, she indignantly told me that she was the one who should be doing those "wifely" things for him. I agreed and the next time it was necessary, I insisted she take care of him. She could not even coordinate her thoughts or her hands enough to do what was required and this only served to anger Dad and to frustrate her further.

For the most part Dad's mind stayed pretty clear. The grandchildren were always a source of joy for him and he never failed to put up a cheerful front for them and play with them until the very last few days.

Ed Spalding, one of our associate pastors, was such a blessing to Dad during those weeks. Before he became bedfast, sometimes Ed would take him to the nursing home to sing and to play the piano for the residents. He was well received by people there. He missed so much sharing his talents with a congregation. Music was also his way of praising and praying. He was gifted with the talent of being able to play anything requested of him and this pleased the residents.

After he became unable to be up, he would often ask me if we were going to put him in the hospital or nursing home. My reply was always, "No, not as long as I can physically, emotionally, and adequately care for you here in our home. But we want to do what is best for you and what will make it easiest for you." This seemed to satisfy him. I think he trusted me and knew I had given him an honest answer as best I could.

7

I Must Not Lose Control! His Grace Must Be Sufficient!!

How does one help another to die? *I don't know!* But we were soon to find out. At an undetermined moment, it seemed that death moved into our house and the regular routine of our happy home life moved out for a time. Death was in charge, once it made its presence known. Death was now calling the shots, planting fear of the unknown in our hearts. Death made it clear that we should make no plans for tomorrow, next week, and maybe even next month. Death reduced activities to those things related to Dad and Mama, such as laundry, cooking, and the little cleaning that must be done. I felt pulled by those church responsibilities that I had assumed months ago and that were now going undone, as well as my pressing home duties. The look of concern and helplessness on the faces of friends who came to call (and who often brought a welcomed dish of food) told us that death had already moved into the guest bedroom on the south side of the house.

Each time Ted visited terminally ill persons as their pastor and friend, he was reminded of his own father's grave condition. Each funeral he conducted reminded him of what was to come. Throughout our ministry we have been near death. As the children were growing up and they inquired about the whereabouts of their dad, for me to say that he had a funeral or had gone to the funeral home was no more to them than to say he had gone to the store. It is such a commonplace occurrence in a minister's home. The fact that there had only been two other close deaths in the Sisk family, Granny and Grandpa Sisk, also made us feel the impact of what was ahead for all of us. Even Granny Sisk used to pray that God would soon come and take her home to be with Him, because she had more waiting for her over there than she had left here. For my family, the Daltons, death had visited more often and taken closer family members. But this too would pass!

Death that makes its presence known and then seems to hang on in suspense, must be the cruelest kind. Our wonderful family doctor, Adam Miller, ignored his own terminal illness and continued to care for Dad. I remember the last time he came to the house. It was a lovely February Saturday morning. The sun streamed through my east kitchen windows and brought a sense of warmth to my soul as well as to the room. Ordinarily my spirits would have been lifted but not today. Adam was so ill himself with cancer that I feared he would collapse in my kitchen. He held so tightly to the back of a chair that his knuckles turned white from the pain. I recall asking if I should call him to come when Dad died and he replied that it would not be necessary but just to let him know and he would sign the death certificate. I thought, *Surely, I am not hearing myself correctly saying these things. I am a person of hope, but here are two people I'm close to who are dying of the same disease. Oh, God, please let this pass from us and be only a dream*! But I knew it would not! Is this helping Dad to die? Yes, we all helped him to die with dignity. Dr. Miller prescribed a strong medication that is so often necessary with cancer patients to ease some of their pain. Thank God, Dad only required one dose.

Months before, we had been told that the doctors had done all they could do for Dad. Ted and Ruth had agreed that they would not consent to a life-support system just to keep him alive when there was no hope for more quality time.

Doctors and nurses are bound by the Hippocratic oath to prolong life, whether or not there is quality; families are not. We wanted Dad to die with dignity, surrounded by those who had loved and cared for him. The only thing we had agreed on was that if it was necessary for him to have oxygen and it could not be administered at home, then we would take him to the hospital.

The night before, we feared we would lose Dad before daybreak. Hardly had we settled down when we heard the labored breathing through the monitor lent to us by our neighbors, the Fowlers. They had only recently experienced this trauma when Betsy's mother had died.

The spot on Dad's lung looked as if it might break through the skin at any time. Dr. Miller had warned that it might erupt. The cancer had now taken over both lungs. If it should erupt, what should I do? How will I handle it myself? Should I tell him, or Mama who would probably become hysterical? "Oh, Heavenly Father, give me wisdom to deal with such as this—I'm not so strong and capable as I thought I was!"

The stench was terrible. No amount of bathing and spraying could take away the odor of death that had moved in. In fact, the whole house smelled like all too many nursing homes. I was sick of the smell of death, urine, and feces! I was sick physically from fatigue. No wonder a friend who brought food over was startled when I opened the door and she said I looked like death myself. I was confused and afraid. Not of death itself but fearful I might be unable to handle all this and keep Dad in our home until he died. The hospital bed helped some with the lifting and less bending, but my bones ached from fatigue.

I found myself running to the Psalms as my refuge for a few moments at a time. I have read the Psalms and parts of them many times, but never in all my life have I read them in light (or should I say darkness) of death as I did then. My copy of *The Living Bible* bears witness to this fact as I underscored verses that ministered to my heart in those days.

Oh, Lord, hear me praying; listen to my plea, O God my King, for I will never pray to anyone but you. Each morning I will look to you in heaven and lay my request before you, praying earnestly (5:1-3).

Pity me, O Lord, for I am weak. Heal me, for my body is sick, and I am upset and disturbed. My mind is filled with apprehension and with gloom. Oh, restore me soon (6:2-3).

All those who know your mercy, Lord, will count on you for help. For you have never forsaken those who trust in you (9:10).

Lord, why are you standing aloof and far away? Why do you hide when I need you the most? (10:1)

Even when walking through the dark valley of death, I will not be afraid, for you are close beside me, guarding, guiding all the way (23:4).

The one thing I want from God, the thing I seek most of all, is the privilege of meditating in his Temple, living in his presence every day of my life, delighting in his incomparable perfections and glory (27:4).

O Lord, have mercy on me in my anguish. My eyes are red from weeping; my health is broken from sorrow. I
am pining away with grief; my years are shortened, drained away because of sadness (31:9-10).

Lord, how long will you stand there, doing nothing? (35:17)

I am too distressed even to pray! (77:4).

The entire Ninetieth Psalm was and is one of my favorites.

His loved ones are very precious to him and he does not lightly let them die (116:15).

Lord, deal with me in lovingkindness, and teach me, your servant to obey;. . . therefore give me common sense to apply your rules to everything I do (119:124-125).

When I pray, you answer me and encourage me by giving me the strength I need (138:3).

These are just examples of the wonderful strength I received from the Psalms.

8

Honest Prayers from a Burdened and Weary Heart

My prayer life became different. I have always felt that God deserved my undivided attention. At least most of the time when I prayed, He got it. My favorite place was to kneel before the den couch. Admittedly, I have had wonderful experiences with the Lord while I was driving the car on a trip alone, or over the ironing board, ironing the numberless shirts that a mother has to in a household with five males of varied shapes and sizes. Some of my prayertime has been humming while I cooked dinner, especially my praise prayers, while I enjoyed the beauty of the late afternoon amidst the sounds of children at play. I realized how good God has been to me and mine through another day, as children left for school that morning and a husband left to do battle with the satanic forces that appeared in various forms through the day. A minister's battle so often is not physical but mental and emotional.

Now that death had moved in, things changed. I caught myself praying on the run. When I knelt to pray my heart would be too full, and I could not utter words though I felt I must—or I would fall asleep from fatigue. My mind went back to the Scripture passages that talk about the Holy Spirit's making intercession for us and how He prays for us "with groans that words cannot express" (Rom. 8:26, NIV) . Then there were those times when I knew I needed to pray but a certain rebellion rose within me and I almost refused to pray.

There were times when I cried out, "Hey, wait a minute, God! This is more than I bargained for! Sure, I vowed at the marriage altar 'for better or for worse, in sickness or in health' but I don't recall any vows about the sickness and death of my in-laws!" Then, I would be overcome with such guilt. Could I not remember the times when they had cared for me and my newborn son so untiringly? Surely there were times when it was not convenient for them to drop everything and run to my rescue but I had taken that for granted. Weren't good mothers-in-law supposed to do that? After all, my own mother was gone and she was the only mother I had—Mama owed me that! I had been a good wife to their son and a good mother to their grandchildren, hadn't I? Yes, I was grateful but I needed to be reminded.

"But Lord, must I be reminded in this way? I am not used to dealing with death and suffering in this fashion. It has always been just enough removed, just far enough away for me to be able to deal with it in a sophisticated manner—the preacher's- wife manner. You know, Lord, just the right amount of sympathy and emotion for people to notice how much I care but not involved enough to lose sleep or get my hands dirty. Remember, Lord, how I've always wanted the parishioners to think I was so able and strong —and capable, too? Am I not supposed to be able to counsel, lead primary organizations, give heartwarming devotions, pray beautiful prayers, lead prayer meetings in the pastor's absence, visit in the homes and hospitals, have perfectly disciplined children, entertain the entire church beautifully, and always look just right? I must not be overdressed or too stylishly dressed but fashionable enough they won't be ashamed of me. I must remember everybody's name and always smile.

"You know, too, Lord, how I like for them to say how wonderful I am to care for my father-in-law in this distasteful situation. Father, who do I think I am fooling? I hate this! I hate the facade I am trying to wear!

"I hate the stench! I hate the spilled urine and coffee on my bedroom carpet. I hate the dust and cobwebs, the packed-up furniture to make room for a hospital bed. I hate the ache in my legs when I climb the stairs countless times. I hate the way I look when

I pass a window and see my reflection, or stand before a mirror to put on enough makeup so that others will not mistake me for a corpse.

"Lord, can't You see what this is doing to me? Old age is chasing me and I am stumbling trying to outrun her. I don't really care how my hair looks. The trip to the beauty shop is too much. I am afraid to leave Mama and Dad alone even for just that couple of hours. What if he should die while I am gone? I would never get over the guilt. Mama staggers and is so unsteady on her feet—they are so swollen. If she should fall down those stairs, he couldn't help her. No, I can't leave them. But who will sit for me?

"I am afraid at night that she will get up to go to the bathroom and fall down the stairs. If we put up a barrier sufficient to keep her from falling, what would we do in the event of fire, if we panicked and couldn't remove it? Besides, I've had enough of a scare about fire when I forgot the meat I was cooking and left the unit on high and went up to give Dad his bath and it caught fire. You know it was Your tender care that kept me from burning the house down then. I shudder to think how next to impossible it would have been to get them out of a burning house into the freezing weather outside. Even after calling the fire department, I couldn't get rid of the smoke and burned smell. I thought I was going to have a heart attack myself when I saw the flames. I wonder what my blood pressure was in that moment of fear with Mama screaming down to me from upstairs that something was burning. Strange how alert she could be at times and how confused at others.

"Where is my own family? Sure, they have their own lives to live. Besides, they don't understand, though I like to think they care. Where is Ruth? These are her parents, too, Lord! Of course, she has had a hard time before with them but could it have been this bad? Does she really think that saying, 'Call me, if you need me,' is enough? Does that relieve her of feeling any responsibility? Hearing her say that doesn't take care of that mountain of dirty sheets and other laundry. It doesn't wash any dishes, vacuum any floors, run any errands, bathe sick bodies, or make me get more hours of sleep.

"Forgive me, Lord, what did I expect her to say? What did I expect her to do? She has family responsibilities, too. Would I really lie down if she came? I have become so attuned to Dad's needs now, would I trust his own daughter to care for him? She hadn't heard the doctor's instructions on caring for him and now he is used to me.

"Lord, I am Your rebellious child! Even though I want to have my own way most of the time, I also want You to be in control—I think.

"Father, I long for those days gone by when Mama and Dad would come and we would talk and laugh and he would entertain us all on the piano and with his tall stories of his own escapades. Remember how the boys would sit and listen with big eyes and unbelieving ears? Often they would say, 'Do that again, Granddaddy!' I long for the happy family gatherings around the big dining room table at 426 West Doyle Street. I regret the wonderful memories I have of the former days will not be so indelibly planted in the minds of my children and grandchildren as they are in mine and Ted's. Lord, let me draw from those former days memories and strength to get me through this.

"Oh, how much I want to bring back those days of seeing Dad enjoy 'sopping' the hot biscuits and gravy or biscuits and my homemade strawberry jam. Once again, I want to see him stir the sugar and cream in his coffee with that crooked little finger sticking out and hear him tentatively refuse a second helping of something that was his favorite, until I insisted that he take it, then see him relish it only to complain that he was eating too much. I want to hear him say to me, 'Honey, you don't need to fix nothing for Mama and me, just bread and jelly will do,' but knowing all the time he was hoping that I would go ahead and fry that chicken and make those biscuits and gravy.

"Jesus, about this feeling in the pit of my stomach—sometimes it is like nausea and I feel I am going to throw up. You know,

Lord, how I like things to be clean and to smell good. Like my mother used to say when I was a child, 'Cleanliness is next to godliness!' Lord, if one of the effects of Alzheimer's disease is incontinence, could that please come later on? I can't cope with that too right now. Please deliver Mama from that indignity. She, too, is suffering so much.

"Oh, I feel like I am pregnant. Oh, please not that now! I am sorry, Lord, but I can't wash and clean that prosthesis. Teach me, Lord! Help me not to throw up, please. Why can't Mama have mind enough right now at least to do that for him? Must I do everything for everyone?

"Hey, Lord, when can I think of myself again? Just me! But I do remember that You have said You would never put more on us than we can bear. Yes, Lord, I can wash the dentures and the prosthesis! Of course, I can—I think! But I am not sure that I can swab out that cavity in his face. Help me, Jesus! I must not get sick! There are too many depending on me. Father, please give me strength for whatever this day holds.

"Lord, is Ted aware of what I am going through? In fact, is anybody aware or caring how I feel? Now, the weather has closed in and a lot of snow is predicted. If we need an ambulance, could it drive up this steep hill? Tonight, Ted will have to move cars up on the driveway so we can be assured of being able to get around tomorrow.

"Lord, You have said you know what I have need of even before I ask, so surely You already know all the things I have just told You. Could I just remind You, Jesus, that we do need Your strength—especially Ted, Mama, and me. We need Your spiritual undergirding for our bodies and our spirits."

It became very easy for me to pray, "Even so, Lord Jesus, come now and take Dad home to be with You. We want him to be free from his suffering and be whole and happy again." I would hear him praying for mercy. I would see Mama sitting crying and yet not fully understanding the gravity of the hour. She would frequently ask me, "He's not going to make it, is he?" I would have to reply honestly, "No, he isn't, but God's strength is sufficient for all of us and Dad will be so much better off." I would remind her that he would be free of his disease and distorted looks. Even in her confused state she would agree and we both knew that we were weeping not for Dad but for ourselves.

9

"Swing Low, Sweet Chariot, Coming for to Carry Me Home!"

Slowly, by experience and acquired knowledge I am beginning to realize that death is as natural to this life as birth. Our youth-oriented society belies this fact. It seems very difficult for us in the prime of life and in great health to think about the possibility of death, much less to consider our own or that of a special person in our lives. When everything is coming up right and we have dreams of love and success, it is hard to face head-on the possibility of death. We have been conditioned from early life to be sad over something dying, whether it is a family pet or a closely watched seed that came up and then died. When things are well, we want it to go on forever. Rarely, under very unusual circumstances, would a youth or young adult pray for someone to die. Why, it would be considered a sin or a curse!

Yet, there are times in our lives when we can pray for the mercy of death. If one has seen living death, as I have, it becomes easy to pray for the release from this life of a loved one caught in the grip of cancer or Alzheimer's disease. I came to know that it was the merciful, gracious thing to do and even to say, "How long, O Lord, how long?"

When I was fourteen, I experienced the death of my own thirty-seven-year-old mother from uremic poisoning during childbirth. I lost my father with heart disease in 1970, but I was not there to help him die. It happened so suddenly. So it seemed as if almost overnight the possibility of my father-in-law's death was staring us in the face, though it was several years before he died.

At the time of Dad's death, we lived in a two-story house. As long as Dad possibly could we let him climb the stairs back and forth to his bedroom. This gave him a sense of independence and encouraged him to keep moving. However, the time soon came when he could not come down so we began taking his meals to him. He was spending less and less time out of bed. Each day we could see a deterioration in his condition. He was consuming fewer liquids and almost no food. He did not want to be hospitalized, and we honored his request. We got a hospital bed for him and moved Mama's bed into the study, the room next to his.

The last three weeks of Dad's life, we realized we had turned our home into a hospice. We were preparing ourselves to help him die. We openly and frankly told him we feared this was the beginning of the end, when he asked us. He would ask how long he had to live, to which we could honestly reply that we did not know, but in our hearts we knew it could not be long. He was naturally obsessed with the prospects of dying. He did not seem to be fearful but more anxious about Mama than himself. We assured him that we would all do our best for Mama. Often I would silently ask the Lord to please make his homegoing easy and as pain free as possible.

On one occasion he asked me point-blank what I thought it would be like to die. He said, "When I die, do you think I am going this way, or that way?" as he moved his hands up and down and from side to side. Surely the Lord gave me this answer. I told him, of course, I didn't know, but I had a little story I wanted to share with him.

"One time there was a little boy who was afraid to go to sleep in his own bed in his room. So he asked if he could go to sleep in his daddy's big bed. His dad said he could and so he did. Then, when the little boy was sound asleep, his father picked him up and took him to his own little bed. When he awoke, he was in his own bed. It was morning and the sun was shining brightly outside. The dew on the grass and flowers looked like sparkling diamonds."

I told him that I believed dying would be just like that; we would go to sleep down here and then Jesus would pick us up in His arms and take us to heaven and when we awoke, we would find ourselves in our own room in heaven. I asked Dad, "Did you like my story?" He just smiled with his eyes closed and said, "Yeah, I like that!"

How can we help one die? Dying should be as natural as birth and no more to be feared for those who have trusted Jesus and committed their life and eternity to Him. Dad had made this commitment years ago when he was a boy, and it seemed that all his life he had been preoccupied with the prospects of heaven and eternal life. Most of the songs that he wrote through the years bore this out. He could have died a wealthy man in dollars and cents had he known how to take advantage of his copyrights and not let others cheat him, but he was a trusting man who was too generous for his own good. Instead, he died a poor man with a song in his heart. Notice the frequent references to life after death in the lyrics of some of his songs.

He wrote many songs. Let me share some of the words and titles that he wrote and set to music. Some of his best-known and loved were "When I Rest on the Bosom of My King," "Press On, It Won't Be Very Long," and "Far Above the Starry Sky," from which the following lyrics stir my soul.

Soon I'll leave this world of sorrow,
For that homeland of the soul,
It will be a bright tomorrow,
When the pearly gates unfold;
Savior, be Thou ever near me,
Till I reach my home on high,
Where I'll rest from all my labor
Far above the starry sky.

Soon I'll walk the streets of glory.
Meet with loved ones gone before,
O what shouting, O what singing,
When He opens wide the door;

Christ Himself will come to greet me,
To that happy home on high,
He will give to me a welcome,
Far above the starry sky.

Come and go with me to glory,
From all sorrow we'll be free,
Then we'll sing love's grand old story,
Just across the jasper sea;
With my harp and crown I'll ever,
Play the song "sweet by and by,"
With the hosts of heaven joining,
Far above the starry sky.

The last song he wrote and published was "Outer Space," The last verse of that song says,

The heav'nly choir will then begin to sing,
In tones that blend with bells that peal and ring
We shall forever there His name adore,
Where time and space will count, no, nevermore.

It will be joy, exceedingly great joy,
There with our Lord, where nothing shall annoy
We'll sing His praise with loved ones gone before,.
Where time and space will count, no, never more.[1]

One of the most precious memories I have of Dad's homegoing is the day our associate pastor came by to visit and pray with him. It was very evident that Dad could not hold on much longer. Ed has a wonderful gentle way with older people and children. After sharing some Scriptures and visiting a little, Ed asked if he could pray. Dad was so choked up he could only squeeze Ed's hand. Then Ed prayed and when he finished, Dad began to pray. It was then my turn and Ed's to be choked up. I shall never forget Dad's praying for others and then asking God to help him do His will. He just kept on praying and praying. Finally, Ed began to say "Amen," but Dad seemed not to notice, so he kept on praying aloud until finally he, too, said "Amen." God is so good! Indeed, He does answer prayers. Sometimes He answers even those prayers we are fearful He won't.

On a dreary, dark February day, the nurse from the county health department had come by. It was evident to both of us that Dad was growing weaker as he only had a bite or two of gelatin and almost no liquids that day. The nurse helped me bathe him and put in a catheter. The stench was terrible and the nurse cautioned me that the place in his lung was about to break to the outside. I felt nauseated thinking *What will I do if it does break through? What if he starts to hemorrhage? Suppose I am downstairs? What will I tell him is happening? This will only make him more anxious! Oh, Lord God, please don't let this happen, take him on home first!*

By the time we got him bathed, the bed changed, and the catheter in, Dad was worn out completely and the nurse was aware of this. She told me that was all he could take for that time and she would be back the next day to do some other things and to check on the dark spot on his rib cage. All the time we were doing these things for him, he was fussing at us. In fact, the last words I ever heard him speak were, "If you two women don't stop, you are going to kill me!" The nurse left and I went downstairs to begin dinner preparation, leaving Mama to sit with him and to call me if he needed something. He seemed already to be sleeping. He was worn out and we had given him a dose of the high-powered medication to control the pain.

As I rushed down the stairs, I remembered that Ted had a meeting at the church so I'd have to fix something quickly and my weary body told me I was too tired to do much more. Fortunately, there were leftovers—that would be a start. Before dinner was ready Ted came in and inquired about his dad. I reported all that had gone on that afternoon but that he was now sleeping, so Ted didn't go up at that moment.

When I had dinner on the table, I asked Ted to check on his dad and bring his mother to dinner. When he came to the door of the bedroom, Dad appeared to be sleeping. Ted did not speak, but motioned for Mama to come. We had a nice, relaxing dinner and sat at the table to exchange the news of activities of the day until Ted had to leave for his meeting. Mark went to his room to begin studying while I started the dishes and cleanup. Before Ted went to the church, he took his mother upstairs and looked in on his dad once more. He appeared to be sleeping.

Before I had finished in the kitchen, Mama came back down the stairs and said, "Will you come check on Theodore? He is so still." I can't describe the almost electric-like shock that went coursing through my body. I knew right then, *This is it!* I can't tell you why I knew that, but my forehead broke out in a cold sweat, and my hands were trembling as I raced upstairs leaving Mama to climb up alone. When I entered the room, he was lying just as he was when I went down nearly two hours before. Not one wrinkle had changed in the bed, his head was in exactly the same position. I bent down low to hear his breathing which was usually very audible—no sound. I checked his pulse— nothing. By then, Mama had gotten back upstairs and was by my side saying, "He's all right, isn't he?" I could honestly say, "Yes, my dear, he is all right now—he has gone to be with the Lord. He is free of pain and cancer. He may even be singing one of his songs with the angels." She didn't comprehend, bless her heart. I said, "Mama, he is dead!" She broke down and her confusion was now compounded by grief that she really could not fathom. I thought of what the apostle Paul said, *I have fought a good fight, I have finished my course.*

I went to the top of the stairs to call Mark. He came and I asked him to go to the church to tell his dad. He later related to me that he had driven furiously, though it was unnecessary now. Ted said to me when he came home, "I thought I had worked through all this and had wept enough but when Mark came and called me from my meeting and told me, I still experienced the knot in my stomach and the tightness in my throat, as my body was wracked with sobs. I guess one is never totally prepared, even for the inevitable. I returned to the room and shared the news with my committee. It was a rare and wonderful privilege to hear those devout friends lift us all in prayer. Two Scriptures, 'Precious in the sight of the Lord is the death of his saints' and 'Blessed are the dead who die in the Lord' came to my mind. My open grief soon gave way to rejoicing."

In a loving, caring church, word spreads fast. It was no time at all before neighbors and friends had come in and put our house back together again as if nothing had ever happened. The hospital bed was removed, the dishes finished, and preparations were begun to make the long trek to Georgia to bury our Dad.

How do people get through the rough times of life without the help of the Lord and His people? I must say a word about the supernatural strength that is ours to draw on in difficult times like these. The Lord did promise us that He would never put more on us than we could bear and that His grace would be sufficient for every trial. Perhaps our minds and bodies can endure more than we think. In my own mind and heart, there were mixed feelings—relief that Dad was at last out of his suffering; sadness that we no longer had him; and fear about what the future held for all of us. One of the great heartbreaks through it all was Mama. Though she had Alzheimer's disease, there were times when she was very lucid and felt the loss of what had happened. Then there were other times when it was obvious she did not comprehend all that was going on. Some of the friends in their hometown seemed unacquainted with the symptoms of Alzheimer's disease. At the wake, I remember one woman in particular who refused to tell Mama who she was, teasing her. Of course, Mama couldn't remember. I interrupted the conversation to say to the lady, "Please tell Mama who you are, she is under a great deal of strain now, and sometimes she doesn't remember too well." Frankly, I was angry that anyone could be so insensitive. Ruth and I had tried to make sure that some family member was with Mama at all times to give her support and answer questions for her. She usually handled her memory loss beautifully. She would just smile and offer her hand. Perhaps most people knew of her problem.

We wish now that we had had a funeral in Lexington before we took the body to Georgia. Our church family had been so support-ive and helpful during this long ordeal. A motor home filled with deacons plus several cars made that long 800-mile round trip to Georgia in terrible, terrible weather to attend the funeral. In fact, the weather was so bad the following day our entire family was snowed in at my brother's house and could not return to Kentucky until two days later. That much snow is so unusual in Georgia that the roads could only be cleared by a regular dirt road scraper, which doubled as a snowplow. Fortunately, a friend with a four-wheel-drive vehicle brought in food and needed supplies .

Theodore Roosevelt Sisk, Sr. was buried a few feet away from his father and mother and his paternal grandparents (under the shade of an old cedar tree) in the old Zebulon Cemetery, on High-way 123, near the city limits of the little town of Toccoa, Georgia.

Part II:

No End in Sight

10

The Way We Were

"You are mighty sure you're going to get him, aren't you?" said Lena Sisk as she watched me monogram a big "S" on a pair of cutwork pillowcases I was finishing for my hope chest. It was a popular thing for a young girl to begin a hope chest when she considered herself a prospective bride. Being the smart aleck I was prone to be, and perhaps being more than a little defensive, my quick retort was, "I tell you what, if I don't get him I'll give the pillowcases to you!" Since I was engaged to her son officially, with a diamond on my left hand, I felt justified and assured of my position to monogram pillow cases, towels, sheets, or whatever I chose with an "S." This was the kind of chiding and teasing that Lena did as she was getting across her point that nothing is really assured until vows are exchanged. I did not feel there was any hidden message in her remark, but neither did I want her to feel she had "put me in my place." So from the very beginning our relationship as mother-in-law and daughter-in-law was good and open—no hidden agenda. We didn't agree on everything, but neither of us felt necessarily obligated to do things exactly the way the other did. In other words, we were free to be ourselves and do things our way.

Perhaps I, too, would have felt somewhat threatened if a teenage girl was making plans to marry my son, even if I had agreed to this engagement. What mother would not have felt that way? I can imagine she was thinking how few years she had had this son who was not through college and did not have a job. Since then, I have experienced some of those same emotions, seeing my sons marry young and then struggle to prepare themselves for their life's work. Come to think of it, she was a pretty well-composed lady. Perhaps she, too, was marveling at the reckless abandon of youthful lovers who were so confident of the future, though Ted had to borrow money from his grandfather to buy modest rings for me. All in all, I have to say that Lena Sisk gave her promising young son to another woman with more grace and love than most of us can. I loved her for that!

One could never say that this tall, handsome lady had had an easy life. She had not. Her own mother had died when she was just nine. She was one of seven children born to Bob and LeNora Smith and fourth from the oldest.

The Smith family were farmers and "lived off the land" until a huge hailstorm destroyed everything planted and there was nothing left to live on. It was then that Bob Smith, a young widower with six children, moved to the little town of Toccoa, Georgia, and began to eke out an existence by working in the textile mills. The housekeeping and child rearing were left to Lena and Grace, the only girls in the family. Things were so bad financially that Grace soon went to work in the mill. At that time younger children were allowed to do that kind of work. This left all the housework and child care to Lena. She attended school as she could but never really had a formal education, though I considered her to be an educated woman. Life had taught her many hard lessons no textbook ever could have.

When Lena's mother died, the older children made their father promise that he would never marry again, and foolishly he promised. His only surviving child today says it was the biggest mistake his father ever made and the most selfish thing his children could have asked of him. The children needed a mother, and his father needed a wife. Ironically enough, after his children left home Bob Smith lived a lonely, unfulfilled life in rented rooms and eventually died alone in a boardinghouse. But a man's "word was his bond" in those days so, painful as it was, he had kept his foolish promise to his selfish children. Mama felt this keenly and would have loved to have taken him into her own home except she did not have "her own" home since they lived all those years with the elder Sisks. Unfortunately, Jesse Sisk and Bob Smith had little love and respect for each other and when Bob would come to visit his daughter and grandchildren, Jesse would ask him almost immediately, "Well, Bob, how long you planning on staying this time?" One could hardly call that rolling out the red carpet! He never stayed more than two or three days. Ted and Ruth loved to have him come because he was fun and was easy to talk to and play with—the exact opposite of Grandpa Jesse.

After Lena married Theodore Sisk and the other children married, Bob Smith moved to Greenville, South Carolina, to work in the textile mills. Most of his other children also moved to Greenville but he did not live with any of them.

By virtue of her early home responsibilities, Mama knew so much when she married. She held the purse strings. She was the frugal one, the manager of the assets, and many times she was the decision maker. It was good that she could manage money because Dad certainly did not. In his younger days, he was not too concerned about money. This was understandable because Grandpa Jesse had told him years before, "You write the music and take care of the music business; I'll make a living on the railroad for all of us." But we all know that the one who makes the money also makes the decisions about how it is spent, and Grandpa Jesse was not always generous as was Theodore. Since this was the way Grandpa insisted it be, it was like a necessity for Theodore not to record every cent that came in from the sale of songbooks and songs he wrote—hence his spending money.

Mama sewed for herself, Ruth, Ted, Granny, and even her granddaughters later on. She loved crafts and made many now-cherished things, such as afghans, tablecloths, and pillowcases, for Ruth and me. She had an eye for beauty and loved her garden club and the prize-winning flowers she often grew. I am the fortunate recipient of much of her expertise in cooking, sewing, and house-keeping. When I make pear preserves, I remember it was she who taught me how as we gathered pears from the old gnarled tree by the music house. Often we had to get the ladder and shake the tree. The music house accommodated the music business on one end and the other end was the washhouse before they got an automatic washing machine for the kitchen. Working with her in the kitchen or out in the yard was not like work at all but play. I drew from her the strength and instruction I would have from my own mother had she lived. I was eager to help her clean closets and drawers—they held so many goodies and mementos from the past.

Granny Sisk never threw anything away. I remember one clean-ing spree I went on in that old house when I threw away Christmas cards that were more than thirty years old. From then on, if some-one couldn't find something in that house, the comment was, "Well, I guess Ginny threw it away with all that other stuff she threw out!" I got the feeling at times that I was not too popular with the older Sisks.

I greatly admired both Lena and Etta Sisk. Not many women can live under the same roof year after year and their relationship remain intact. There were times when how intact it may have been was questionable. Each admired the other and realized they needed each other, but they didn't always see eye to eye. I have tried to imagine myself in each one's place and I have had real difficulty—and I have some wonderful daughters-in-law. As the years came and went, it became more and more Lena's house. This came about partly because of Granny's advancing age but also be-cause she admired the way Lena did things like cooking and sew-ing. Granny was content to do the darning and mending, sweeping the front porch and walks, bringing in the wash from the line, stringing the beans and shelling the peas, or washing up where someone else cooked. But in earlier years it was Granny who cared for Mama and new babies as if she were her own daughter. Indeed Mama was the only daughter Granny had. It was Granny who prescribed home remedies for all the family, who prayed for each one as if it all depended on her and her faithfulness to pray. It was also Granny who complained a lot but really loved every minute of it. When she was waiting on someone else, especially Lena, she was in charge again and making decisions. She was the queen bee once again.

But all the giving and compromising was not just on Granny's side. I have tried to imagine moving into the house with another woman and having nothing of my own but having to keep house with her things, doing things her way. Having entered into a marriage without parental blessing must have added to the tension that existed between two good, strong-willed women. They learned to live together and although each did things that irritated the other, still each would defend the other. Mama really grew up without a mother from her early childhood years, as did I as a teenager, so Granny filled that void in her life as well.

Mama was not as demonstrative in her love as Dad was, but her devotion, love, and commitment ran deep—it was constant and consistent. Nor was she as excitable and impulsive as Dad was, as a rule.

Case in point! The night Ted was born, Dad was sent to the backyard for something. There was a sheet hanging on the clothesline in the yard flapping in the cold January wind. He was startled by this and ran to get a gun. Aunt Eula, who lived next door overheard him say, "If you make one more move, I'll blow your brains out!" Doubtless, he took a lot of ribbing about shooting the sheet, but he was an impetuous man. How can I be too critical? After all, this was their second baby in thirteen months. Some men might have been tempted to turn the gun on themselves. Having two babies so close together created health problems for Mama. Her doctor encouraged her to "eat for two" therefore, she gained too much weight which she never lost and had other health problems that prevented them from having more children.

Her children have had nothing but the utmost respect for their mother. She has walked before them in the Spirit and lived an exemplary life before them. They saw Proverbs 31 lived out in her.

She was the heavy in discipline while Dad was a pushover most of the time or else he would overdo it. She frequently had to leave the children with Granny and Grandpa Sisk while they were gone for weeks at a time in singing schools or other things related to the music business.

Mama's beautiful voice was a real asset. She once played the organ for what was then Second Baptist Church in Toccoa where she met Theodore; but after she married him she never played again. She felt that as a musician he was so much better than she was. He didn't encourage her to play either since he loved doing it.

Ted and Ruth hated being left while their parents traveled, and everyone felt that Grandpa Jesse was too hard on them and punished them for the slightest offense. Grandpa always wanted to be "cock of the walk" and usually was. Ted and Ruth tell the story of the time when they and the neighbor kids were out on the side lawn playing cards (which was strictly forbidden in that household), when they saw Grandpa approaching from the railroad. He was supposed to be on a long run to Greenville and was not expected home until the next day. They had felt safe playing openly. Since it was too late to run, they decided to continue playing. Grandpa walked up and stood behind Ted to watch, saying not a word until Ted started to play a certain card. Grandpa then nudged him with his knee and said "Uh-uh, Uh-uh!" Then they all knew that Grandpa Sisk knew how to play cards, too. He did not reprimand them this time for playing but turned and made his way into the house. Grandpa felt he had to be hard. After all, he was a Pentecostal Holiness preacher who wore no tie, an autocrat who called all the shots or tried to. Needless to say, there were many times when Mama and Grandpa Jesse butted heads, especially over the rearing of the children. But his domineering way wasn't all bad. Ted speaks fondly and gratefully of the way the entire family was required each night to kneel before worn cane-bottom chairs in Grandpa's bedroom/sitting room (the only room that had a fire in it in the wintertime) and take turns praying after they had read from the *King James Version* of the Bible that lay on the mantel over his fire. Frequently he would take Ted on his knee when he was a little boy and ask, "Son, do you love Jesus?"

Mama hated having only one room besides the kitchen heated because the house was poorly insulated with high ceilings and uncarpeted floors in most rooms. She frequently put bricks or flat irons on the stove in the kitchen while she was cooking supper or near the fireplace to get warm so she could wrap them in paper and a towel and put them in a cold bed for the children. Everyone would sit or stand before the fire to get toasty warm and then run across the hall and jump in bed with the bricks. Mama and Granny made quilts and the beds were piled so high with them that it was difficult to turn over in the night. It made one tired just to sleep under the weight of all those quilts and blankets.

After Grandpa Sisk died, the Sisk Music Company was bought out and Dad became a salesman. Sometimes he sold insurance, sometimes vacuum cleaners and other things. His personality made him a great salesman. Money was not quite so tight since Grandpa did not hold the purse strings. For years Mama had wanted to do some things to the house and replace some appliances with more modern ones. Now she could, but she was still very conscious of spending and saving. Having an electric stove and washing machine in the kitchen was great.

Most holidays we spent with the Sisk family. My large Banks County Dalton family didn't always get together since my grandmother had gotten older and my mother had died. My father remarried only three months before Ted and I were married. A real sense of family existed with the Sisks. I was a frequent visitor in the Sisk house before we were married and especially on holidays. On one of those occasions I remember Mama opening the door to the "front room" which was the living room as we know it today. I was sitting in Ted's lap before the fire. She let us know in no uncertain terms that she did not think that proper behavior for two unmarried people although we were engaged. But that was the end of it and I don't ever recall her bringing it up again. She loved me like a daughter and reprimanded me as such when she felt inclined to do so. I loved her like a mother, as indeed she was!

She was strong in so many ways. Physically she was a big woman, almost six feet tall and carried herself regally. Spiritually, she had a strong, unswerving faith in Christ. She believed the best about people unless she had reason not to. She had deep-seated convictions about her Christian faith, her children, and her politics. She was loyal to her friends and neighbors and instilled in her children a sense of integrity and commitment.

She was capable of defending and fighting for those things and people precious to her. The story is told of a brazen woman who came to her one time and asked her to divorce Dad so she could have him. She minced no words telling this woman off and showing her the door. She included a few threats to boot, just in case this woman had second thouhts about pursuing her quest of taking another woman's husband.

The anticipation of a visit to the Sisk home in Toccoa always brought me warm, cozy, secure feelings. Years before it had been the house that Jesse Sisk coveted when he was a barefoot boy walking the streets of Toccoa. He swore that one day he would own that house and he did. In the years that followed it became many things to many of us.

It was easy to see that the house had been built before the turn of the century. The porch that went halfway across the front and down one side, had a banister with turned spindles and gingerbread work at the top of intermittently placed posts that were symmetrically arranged along the sides. The wooden floor, even though it was painted each spring, had to be replaced ever so often because of exposure to the weather. The front door was a treasure with stained glass surrounding a clear etched panel in the top half. The side panels had the same clear glass but without the etching. Surrounding all of this was an ornate facing that made the entrance distinctive.

One entered a hallway about twelve feet wide which went all the way to the back of the house. From each side each room opened onto the hallway. The only exceptions were the tiny sleeping porch that was once Ted's room and a room off the dining room which appeared to have been added on at the end of the side porch when it was needed. This was Harlan's room until he went to Emory University in Atlanta. Later one end of the sleeping porch was enclosed to make a family bathroom and a tiny screened porch was added at the back where I frequently saw Granny sitting in a short-legged chair to string beans or to mend. The light was good here and shaded in the morning. From the porch, one could see the huge blue hydrangea and the fig and pear trees at each end of the music house. In the wintertime when the trees were bare, it was easy to see Uncle Marion (Grandpa Jesse's brother) and Aunt Eula's house and the fish pond with many goldfish in it.

Each room, except the sleeping porch and Harlan's room, had a fireplace with a grate. The fireplaces were seldom used because of the expense of coal unless someone was sick, of course. This was a very frugal family as were most of their contemporaries. The kitchen had no grate or fireplace but for many years had a wood cooking stove that made that room the coziest of all, especially when a meal was being prepared. To see a churn of milk "turning" behind the stove or to see clothes hung to dry in the winter were frequent sights. Hence, the kitchen with the single light bulb hanging from the ceiling was used not only for feeding the family but for ironing, sewing, doing homework or whatever chores could be done there in cold weather. Everyone gravitated to the kitchen and even after dishes were done, sat around the table playing games. It was a routine thing to have to run people off the kitchen table so Mama could set it for a meal. Meals around this table were usually simple, wonderful country cooking often consisting of just fresh vegetables and dessert. If Grandpa was home, however, there was always meat on the table.

The front room or living room/parlor was on the front of the house and rarely used. It was closed up to stay clean; so in the summer it was cool with its high ceilings and cold painted wooden floors around a square of carpet. The piano was there, and if Dad was writing music, the room got lots of use. This was also the room where piano pupils had their lessons each Saturday. It was in this room that Granny took her prayer partners when they dropped in to pray with her. Even with the hall door closed, one could hear these women calling on the Lord, making intercession for their families. For as long as I can remember, devout women, both black and white, would come and ask Granny to pray with them.

Each year the Christmas tree was in this room in front of the bay windows. After dinner on Christmas Day, a fire would have been built in the grate by Granny and we would exchange gifts. The only times I ever remember seeing Grandpa in this room was on Christmas Day. This really was not a living room but a special room, reserved for special events. Ted and I did a lot of courting in this room so it has special significance for me.

The hall with a high ceiling, like all the other rooms, was later partitioned off to make a den that housed furniture, a television, and a gas floor furnace. At the same time, most all the rooms got a radiant gas heater installed for warmth but no air-conditioning was necessary. In the back hall was an old refrigerator that had a round condenser on top and too little space inside. Shelves, covered with a faded green curtain, lined the back wall holding all the home-canned goods the women had put up during the summer months. Some of my favorites were the pear preserves and the fig preserves from the old fig tree on the opposite end of the music house. The garden plot below the music house provided most of the vegetables.

In the hall, near the front door stood a beautiful antique oak hall tree where hats and coats were hung. The lift-up lid seat hid an assortment of things that seemed never to have an assigned spot, such as games, a magazine someone wanted to keep, a box of greetings cards with stamps, a "good,clean paper sack," rubber bands, and dull pencils. After grandchildren came, a few toys and other odds and ends could be found there.

Near the hall tree on a small, half-circle table was the telephone with a thin, dog-eared Toccoa directory under it. I can still hear Granny, with her lower lip filled with snuff, answer the phone by saying, "Five-eight!" in a long Southern drawl.

Out front and on the side of the house were three or four large Southern magnolias that continually dropped their leaves; but the aroma was delightful. Grandpa had insisted that these trees have their limbs trimmed off so that a tall man could walk under them and so that someone rocking on the front porch could see the neighbors coming up the street. This meant that every dropped leaf showed and had to be raked. When Ted was a boy, this was his assigned chore, and he learned to hate it. Little wonder that we do not have magnolias in our yard now.

In the side yard of the house, which was really another lot, were several growing things, including a cactus that had been brought back from a trip to Texas. In this side yard grew the flowers that became specimens at the garden club, especially the award-winning irises and day lilies.

Years before, a tiny car house (not called a *garage* then by this family) was built to protect the first car owned by the Sisk family. The house was just barely large enough to get a car in and close the door. By the time I came into the family, cars had gotten larger and the "car house" was in disrepair and not being used as a garage but more as a toolshed. It opened onto Oak Street and was later torn down after Grandpa Jesse died.

It was in this setting that Lena Smith Sisk began her married life, brought her children into the world, and raised them. Hardly an enviable position for most American women today.

Mama had a lovely alto voice when she married Dad, but with his coaching and her maturity, it became even more melodious and sweet. She was a full partner in their gospel-music ministry as they traveled all over the South. Hearing her sing "I Won't Have to Cross Jordan Alone" as a solo would bring tears to the eyes of worshipers. To hear her join Dad as they sang "I'll Meet You in the Morning" would bring people to their feet in applause. As the two children got older and joined the group, making a quartet, they were a very popular group in Southern churches. But as Ted and Ruth left for college, other arrangements had to be made for people to replace them. It was never quite the same again.

Although Mama was a woman of strong character and faith, she was afflicted with hypochondria; she was not the strong one when she was sick. She was never truly healthy after the children were born. One of her favorite expressions was, "I've never had pain like that before in all my life!" She did require some surgeries, so no doubt she was sick a lot but she also had a low threshold for pain. As I describe her to you, I realize I'm getting pretty picky if all I can find to single out as a weakness is hypochondria.

She was known as the Kate Smith of Southern Gospel Music. She sang in the choir of the First Baptist Church, Toccoa, Georgia, and strongly complemented the alto section. She loved her Sunday School class and never missed when she was in town. To attend the daytime Sunday School class meetings was a highlight for her. She never served as an officer other than a group or care leader, but she cherished that relationship.

She was truly a pious woman but did not "go to seed" about it. She was a loving mother who had a tender heart, who held her children close very often, affirming them and encouraging them to be all they were capable of being—striving to be the best. They don't recall ever hearing her use even slang language, much less profanity. She never had a cigarette or a drink of alcohol in her life. Her heart was so tender she could truly "Rejoice with them that do rejoice, and weep with them that weep"(Rom. 12:15, KJV).

Perhaps her closest friend and confidant was Aunt Eula. Among other things, they shared a love of flowers and a garden. Aunt Eula and Granny Sisk were sisters-in-law but very different in their demeanor and outlook on life. Mama's friendship and love for Aunt Eula may have been a source of contention at times between Mama and Granny. Without a doubt, Aunt Eula was the sounding board for many of Mama's frustrations in the early years of her marriage as she struggled to adapt to living in another woman's home, using her things, and trying to be the submissive wife and daughter-in-law at the same time.

She later said that she thought Dad had money of his own when he was trying to persuade her to marry him. He had brought Grandpa Jesse's bankbook down and showed her the balance, which led her to believe that they could afford a place of their own. But they never owned a house of their own. They just rented as they moved out briefly when Dad was working in Atlanta and later when he went to Alexander to serve a church.

11

The Erosion of a Mind

It was one of those crisp November days when the sun was as bright as a freshly washed, sparkling diamond, the kind of day when you want to walk in the woods, kick the leaves, or hear the twigs pop underfoot. Not a cloud in the sky could be seen. This must be my very favorite time of the year but then I remembered that I had said summer with all its floral beauty was my very favorite time of year. I had also said that about spring, when things were coming up and life seems fresh and new—when the resurrection of Christ was so real and believable. I must confess that I always say, "This is my very favorite time of the year," regardless of the season.

Driving home, from the Kentucky Baptist Convention in 1972, after a good, inspirational session was so relaxing. Seeing friends we had met in our last two years in Kentucky was good. At last I had begun to feel at home there after leaving my beloved adopted state of West Virginia.

There seemed so little time to have Ted all to myself and feel good about knowing the boys were well cared for. As we rode along we remarked how fortunate we were to have each other, to have our four wonderful sons, and a family who would drop everything and come to stay with our kids. Mama and Dad really felt they had a part in our ministry by making themselves available to keep the boys so that I could go with Ted and be a relevant partner in his calling. They knew I could not and would not leave them that much with sitters and strangers. Besides, who would want to take on the care of three teenage boys for nearly a week? (Larry was now a sophomore at the University of Cincinnati.)

I knew that when we arrived home at dinnertime there would be a meal on the table and the house would be straight enough. I anticipated a long, leisurely dinner prepared well by this woman I loved as my own mother. Later we would probably play table games until bedtime. We wanted to give this night to Mama and Dad because in all probability they would leave for Georgia in the morning. I could almost smell the fire that would be burning in the den fireplace mingled with the smell of good food.

The boys would be eager to bring us up to date on all that had happened at school since we left. Well, maybe not Jon—he was quieter than the others and also he had a part-time job in the afternoon and evening after school.

When we drove into the driveway, I took the few personal things and went on into the house through the garage. Through the years, Ted has always insisted on loading and unloading the car when we make a trip. When I opened the kitchen door, I saw that the table was only partially set and Mama was standing by the sink crying. Flour was everywhere and the kitchen was in terrible shape. I did not smell the aroma of wonderfully prepared food but instead burned or scorched things. Immediately, I went to Mama asking, "What in the world is wrong—are you sick? Have the boys hurt your feelings? Is Dad all right?" But she could only cry and say, "What is the matter with me? Am I losing my mind? I can't remember how to do anything! I have ruined our supper. Please don't be mad at me—I don't know what's the matter."

As I remember, this was the first inkling we had that something was happening to Mama. She had always been so in control. Admittedly, she was a hypochondriac but we all knew that when the chips were down Mama would come through. At first, I told myself and Ted that her blood pressure probably was high and the week had just been too much for her. After all, taking care of a husband and three teenagers is no small task, especially when one is not accustomed to doing that. The laundry alone at our house would make one's blood pressure rise because the boys could go through clean clothes as if there was no tomorrow. Then, too, I wondered how many other last-minute "guests" my boys had brought home to the dinner table with little or no notice since I had been gone. Being a grandma sometimes makes it hard to say no to grandchildren. It was not uncommon to have one of mine lead a stranger into the kitchen asking if he could eat with us that night.

Whatever was wrong with Mama, I had a deep, frightened feeling it was not simple. To be so out of control like this was not like her.

Looking back now, we believe this was the first evidence we saw of her Alzheimer's disease. I quickly changed my clothes, jumped in, and tried to clean up the mess and fix dinner for all of us. My bubble had burst! There was no fire burning in the fireplace. The sun had now gone down, and the outside chill that was in the air had somehow crept inside and was like a cloud that wouldn't go away. We all tried to be cheerful and reassure Mama. The rest of the evening passed without incident.

The next day as they left for Georgia she seemed like her old self. We all felt relieved and it was easy to push the evening before to the back of our minds and rationalize about it. Later we learned that other things like that were happening. As she grew worse, there were scenes at their church or other public places. After a while we learned that Dad was covering for Mama more and more, making excuses about her behavior. Little did we know then that her housekeeping skills were slipping and she no longer was careful about her own hygiene and appearance. Ironically enough, I remember when I would invite her to go to the grocery with me, her reply would invariably be, "Oh, I'd like to go with you but I need to bathe a little before I go out. Give me just a minute or two!"

Gradually things deteriorated with Mama and Dad. They decided to move to Alexander, Georgia, where Dad would be minister of music for the little Baptist church there. It was a difficult decision for both of them but mostly for Dad. He had lived in the rambling old house in Toccoa for years and years. This was the house where as a teenager he had brought his bride on a cold December night. It was the house where their children had been born and reared—the house Grandpa yearned for as a boy and finally got enough money to buy. It was here that Grandpa had lived his last years and finally died—the house Granny had loved and worked so hard to keep—the house she shared with another woman. It was the house where she, too, had lived until she died.

So much needed to be done to put the house in good living condition, and there just simply was not enough money. The cherished music house was practically falling in, the roof leaked, and the floors creaked. Inside the big house, the walls needed paint, and the floor coverings needed to be replaced. The money that might have been used and was earmarked for such, had to be spent on doctor bills and nurses for Grandpa. A few times Granny had sold land to an unscrupulous buyer who had cheated both her and Dad. They had no idea of the value of land, and they trusted people who actually took advantage of them. So, the house and double corner lot were sold for a pittance and Mama and Dad moved.

Mama decided to sell some of the antiques and other things they could not use where they were going. At the time she had the sale, neither Ruth nor I could be there to help her so once again people robbed her. She had priced things too cheaply in her confusion, not knowing the value of antiques. Even family members and close friends took advantage of her. Many things were actually stolen when her back was turned. So her mental condition, plus her inability to know the value of things, made the sale a disaster benefiting only those who had bought her treasured things. It was good that Granny was not there to see how her beloved things went. It seems the decision to move from Toccoa was made independently of their children.

Not too long after the kitchen scene at our house, Ted was in revival in Augusta, Georgia, near their home. He had bragged to his pastor friend that his mother could cook the best fried chicken and cream gravy in the world. He wanted to take him to have lunch with Mama and Dad. Ted called his mother. Everything seemed fine and the time was agreed upon. All the way over Ted reminisced about his childhood and wonderful tables of food his mother used to prepare.

When they arrived, it was not like he had envisioned at all. The house was not spotless and things did not remind him of his boyhood. He was terribly embarrassed at having brought his preacher friend over. He was also sick to see what had happened to his mother and her appearance. The meal was not ready. It was not well planned and when they finally did sit down to eat, it was hardly edible. The chicken was burned but not done on the inside. The biscuits were horrible and nothing she had fixed was really fit to eat. Dad could only say to Ted, "I don't know what's got into your mother! She don't cook nothing fit to eat any more. I can't cook but I believe I could beat her!" Thus the denial began for all of us for awhile. Sometimes Dad would remark that Mama often acted like she was crazy or losing her mind—she did such goofy things.

Even with all these symptoms, we still assumed it was hardening of the arteries because of high blood pressure. We knew that from time to time she would see a doctor in a neighboring small town. We assumed also that he was keeping check on everything and that he knew her behavior was bizarre and strange. To tell the truth, we sort of chalked it up to her advancing age and her physical condition. At that time, *Alzheimer's* was a new and almost unheard of word to us. It was one of those things that always happened to someone else. Is it not true that we don't want to face up to the fact that our parents do change and have less ability both mentally and physically as they advance in years? Personally, I felt I had already given up a young mother at the time I needed her most, and I didn't want to think about losing this woman who had really taken her place. So I, too, denied it could be serious.

For awhile after they moved to Alexander, Mama seemed to do pretty well. Almost from the beginning, however, we noticed she was different when we visited. At times she would be worse than at other times. She had gotten so indifferent about housekeeping that Ruth and I would take over the cooking and cleaning when we were there. One of the first things we would do would be to wash all the dishes and cooking utensils to remove the greasy film and dust that collected on everything. Frequently, there would be evidence of mice or there would be a problem with ants or roaches. We would find food that had been pushed to the back of the refrigerator and had grown a beard of gray mold, or fruit and potatoes hidden and forgotten until they aroused everyone's attention by their foul odor.

Mama seemed actually relieved when we came to visit and took over. Most women would have objected to a daughter or daughter-in-law doing that, but it was almost as if Mama knew something was badly wrong and she was glad we were doing this for her.

It could hardly be called a vacation when we went to their house in those days. But it was a good feeling to know that before we left we had once again set things in order, cleaned the house, made minor repairs and, hopefully, helped them a little. Dad especially appreciated what we did.

No one could ever accuse Mama of being a fashion plate when it came to clothes, but she always looked nice and had things that were coordinated with the proper accessories. Now that her mind was deteriorating we noticed some unusual combinations. Often her slip would be showing or she would have on a blue and a black shoe. Often she would lose things or rather couldn't find the things she had so carefully hidden. She would forget which dresser drawers were hers so she had clothes everywhere—even in the drawers in the dining room. She would hide her "good" towels that she saved for company and not remember where they were. She often thought people had stolen her things and this scared and disturbed her. She couldn't remember her neighbors' names when they would come to her door. She couldn't remember her own telephone number or what day of the week it was. Little by little Alzheimer's became the thief that stole her memory, her reasoning, and her decision-making ability.

She began to get up in the middle of the night and couldn't find the bathroom, or she would get up to answer the phone that wasn't ringing. Once she fell over a floor fan that was in a doorway and hurt herself by bruising and banging up her legs. This caused sores that would not heal. In retrospect, we know now that her diabetes was very active then.

Eventually, they had to give up their place and job in Alexander and move to Marietta. Only then did we really find out how much Dad had been covering for her, making feeble excuses to others about her condition. For him, it was a denial that this could really be happening to her. By now his own physical condition had reached a climax, and he had had to have radical surgery. In reflecting on the past, I am sure we didn't give Dad the support he needed at this time, but he tried to conceal the gravity of her condition and continually made excuses for her. His impatience with her only aggravated her condition and gave him a sense of defeat and guilt. No one really knows what they went through when they lived by themselves.

Dad often revealed his moods by writing little paragraphs, more for his eyes than others. I recently ran across one and the following paragraph expresses his feelings for Mama at this time in their lives.

"Lena has been a darling wife. She is still sweet to me and I love her so dearly. She has some trouble with her memory but I won't forsake her—I can't do that. She can't remember too well, neither can I, but through all the storms and sunshine we still love each other. Sometimes it is hard to understand but we'll try to, long as we live."

So it was that Mama's household things were boxed up and brought to a strange apartment that would be her last home where the two of them lived alone. I have tried to imagine how devastating it would be to have two of my daughters-in-law to come into my home and take over, deciding what I could take with me and what I could not. What would it be like to be left behind and not even be there to help decide what I could bring to my new place? This is what we did when we moved them to Marietta. This was deliberate because we felt it would be less painful for her and surely quicker since she could no longer make decisions properly. Actually, I doubt that she ever missed any of the things we didn't bring because she could not remember.

Things were set up for them and we hoped that familiar things would help her. But she didn't take much interest in her apartment. She would sit for hours in front of the television watching the "soaps" but being unable to remember what had taken place the day before. I don't think it matters much though, even if one doesn't have Alzheimer's, because often the plot develops so slowly. I never have had that habit, but the few times I have watched, I have the feeling I couldskip a week and still not miss anything.

By now Mama could no longer manage the family funds, remember a telephone message, remember where things were in the house, when she had a bath, or even when she had talked to her children last. She would have better days, and Dad would be encouraged that she was at last "coming out of it." The next day or ever an hour later she might have relapsed into her former sick self. Having conversation with her now was pretty futile. She would ask the same questions over and over, never remembering your answer. It was like a cog on a wheel that would hang onto that peg as it came around each time. We soon learned that it was useless to get upset or even impatient with her because she was not trying to be difficult. Actually, she was probably doing the very best she could. The fault was ours for not being aware of this. Being human as we were, it would sometimes get pretty tedious to answer the same questions over and over.

12

The Longer Road

If I had thought the road was long as we struggled with Dad's surgery for cancer and ultimately his death, I didn't really know anything. At least we knew from the diagnosis and prognosis that he could not be here long in his body wracked with pain and disease. Hard as it is to think or to say—there was light at the end of the proverbial tunnel. With Alzheimer's disease—not so!

At this time, so far as we knew, Mama's blood pressure, arthritis, and other less-threatening ailments were under control. After the official diagnosis of Alzheimer's, we were given little encouragement that she would improve but rather a bleak picture of gradual impairment continuing.

By the time the family concluded that she must have something other than hardening of the arteries and we had sought a professional diagnosis, she had all the classic symptoms. But she was still a master at some things. One was her ability to hide or deny that anything was wrong. Our physician asked her simple questions like her age, her birth date, her mother's name, how many children she had and so on. To each one she would reply to the doctor, "Ginny can tell you" or "Let me think . . ."

After Dad had died, Ted and Ruth agreed that they would each take Mama for a three-month period but living four hundred miles apart made that difficult. She could not travel alone and family members all had home or career responsibilities. Caring for such a person takes a major toll on one. I must confess that the shortest time of my life during those years occurred between the end of

Mama's stay with us and the beginning of the next visit. This was not a good arrangement because Mama could not remember from one day to the next, and each time she moved she could not even remember having been there before. I have sincerely tried to imagine coming into my home and having absolutely no memory that I had ever been there before. Nothing would look familiar! I would not know which toothbrush was mine, so apparently I would figure one is as good as the next one. I could not find the bathroom, and if I did find it I would not know what it was for. So I really would not seek it but would relieve myself of my natural bodily urges where I was.

When a victim is in the advanced stages of Alzheimer's disease, it is not at all uncommon for him or her totally to forget how to use the toilet. Therefore, it is necessary for someone always to go with the victim to prevent him or her from putting their hands and other things in the toilet bowl or making the bathroom totally uninhabitable until major and drastic cleaning has been done. This is an almost unspeakable burden for the caregiver and often precipitates the consideration of other arrangements or facilities for the patient. Therefore, it becomes the responsibility of the caregiver to remember to "take" the victim to the bathroom at regular intervals. Often, this is not sufficient and special undergarments must be used, such as adult briefs or diapers.

The Alzheimer's victim also forgets how to dress—which garments go on first. Often sleeves are mistaken for legs and vice versa. I recall more than once when I had dressed Mama for church on Sunday morning and would have put on makeup (which she loved) and combed her hair, she would redress herself while I was slipping into my dress just before we left. Once I was running late, and Mama had gone back to her room and put on three more slips. It was too late to change and make it to church on time, so I just let her wear them that day. She didn't seem to care, and to me she just looked fat.

Caregivers need help! My husband had to be in Nashville on business and invited me to go with him. I needed a break, so our college-aged son, Mark, agreed that he would look after his grand-mother at night. On the way to classes the next day, he would drop her off at another son's house until I could get her twenty-four hours later. I had taken care of everything—bath, dinner, dressed for bed, explained many times where I was going and that Mark would be there with her all night. It seemed to upset her and she remarked that Mark was just a "kid." (He was twenty years old.) After we left, Mark went to his room to study. When he heard a noise in the kitchen, he went to investigate and found his grand-mother trying to cut her toenails with a butcher knife! He eventu-ally got her to bed but spent a sleepless night keeping an eye on her room for fear she would get up again. We never asked him again to take care of her overnight.

Dinner time in our household has always been an end-of-the-day pleasure. I love to cook. I have an appreciative husband and family. Through the years, the boys have been made to eat some of everything and not allowed to complain about the food. All this makes for a pleasant time at the evening meal. My husband has often said it is with a profound sense of gratitude that he bowed before the Lord at the end of the day to ask the blessing over din-ner and looked around to see our healthy, normal, and very active children after having seen so many in the hospitals suffering or after listening to a sordid story in counseling. All this is to say that dinner time has always been special. It has been a time to share when unexpected guests arrived. Sometimes it meant stretching six pork chops into seven when a son brought a friend in and said, "Mom, can he eat with us tonight?" Frequently, my reply has been, "But I only have six pork chops tonight. Wouldn't another night be better?" Only to have my child reply, "Aw, he can have half of mine . . . please Mom. Please, huh, Mom?"

But alas, all this changed when Mama could no longer remem-ber how to use her knife, fork, or spoon. No longer could we eat family-style with food in serving dishes to be passed. Every plate had to be fixed at the stove and set before each one, or Mama would eat out of the bowls with her hands. Serving the plates was not a complete answer because she would still often reach over and eat from another's plate. No longer could we eat out at a restaurant on Sunday after church. No longer could we accept invitations to friends' homes—or if we did, we had a sitter. No longer could Mama remember that she shouldn't stir or poke at the cooking food. When Alzheimer's victims eat with their hands, that increases the laundry, the floor mopping, and washing the chairs and table. Many of these things most of us never even consider a problem until we are faced with the predicament.

From what I have observed and read, the sense of smell diminishes considerably when persons are stricken with this terrible disease. When the sense of smell goes, so goes the personal hygiene. If they cannot remember when they had a bath and the sense of smell is nearly gone, they are not aware of their need. I personally believe many of the other senses diminish as well. Touch and sight don't seem so keen either. When they are wet they are unaware, or if they are wet often, it becomes the norm rather than the unusual. All of this would seem to suggest that the power of reasoning is also largely gone.

If the power of reasoning is gone, they cannot remember how to peel a banana or an orange. To see a sandwich on their plate is a puzzle how to eat it so why not take it apart bit by bit, or if they still understand using a knife and fork, why should they not try to cut it into bites? I would think *How could she not remember that jelly went on toast instead of eggs?* To eat a baked potato without help was an overwhelming problem. At a certain stage, it might also be embarrassing to have a family member do this for her. How could she know that meat should be cut instead of picked up, or if cut, how could she know that a bite too large might cause her to choke? It is so easy to think, *Surely, she hasn't forgotten that!* None of us can really imagine what it would be like to forget everything—especially the simple things we learned as we were growing up—like how to eat.

Once Mama fell and broke her hip and had to have hip-replacement surgery, but she could not remember falling. She did recognize pain and would say it hurt; but as she progressed and the hip mended, she did not favor it and so her recovery was swift and complete. She did not know or remember that she should be careful. She did not recognize the hospital for what it was and would often ask why she was there and could she go home now. Of course, she was told repeatedly the answers, but in a few minutes it was the same thing over again. She offered no objection when the nurses got her up to walk or took her to therapy. She would say, "I hurt right here!" (pointing to her hip) as she walked.

Rarely did we see her hostile in the least and never hateful. We had been cautioned that as her disease intensified she would probably become very hostile and combative, but we personally never found it so. However, this is not true of most Alzheimer's patients. I have a friend whose mother has Alzheimer's disease. After my friend has been with her mother, she comes away with bad bruises where her mother literally hits her so hard. Her mother, who is a large woman and seems to have super strength, is very uncooperative. Giving her a bath is a major undertaking. It takes more than one person to do this and it is still hard to do. When the primary caregiver is a person of the opposite sex, to do those personal things like trips to the bathroom and bathing can be extremely embarrassing for the patient as well as the caregiver.

One man I know has a mother who is ill with this terribly debilitating disease and whose father is still in the denial and embarrassment stage. He will not let anyone help him bear his load. He only calls on his children for help when there is absolutely no other way. He has devoted his entire life to her now. She is his child that he feeds, dresses, caresses, and looks after. He does the cooking, cleaning, laundry, and everything else required to keep a household going. Much of the time she does not know him. As her mind wanders, she thinks he is first this one and then that one. He bears that hurt all alone by choice. He thinks he is protecting his children from seeing their mother in such a state. Somehow, he must feel that this is part of the "for better or for worse, in sickness and in health" that he pledged himself to years ago when they married. This is admirable to a point, but it is also laying a guilt trip on his children because they know what he is going through alone, and they are shut out. They fear she will outlive him because he is so fatigued all the time.

Once when it was time for a trip to the doctor, the husband of this lady was trying to get her bathed and dressed. She was most uncooperative and stubborn. He could not get her gown off. Because of the approaching time of the appointment and his own fatigue, the husband relented and called his son to come help him. But the son and the husband could not undress the mother to get her ready. After some time, they agreed to let her go in her gown because surely doctors have seen patients like this before. They managed to get her coat on, and off they went. It was the best they could do. Sometimes forcing the Alzheimer's patient to do some things can be very exasperating, because of the clouded mind of the patient. Incidents such as this take their toll on both mind and body of the caregiver.

In earlier stages of Alzheimer's disease there are things that patients can do. Of course, whatever they can do they should be allowed to in order to make them feel useful and independent as long as possible. For example, taking a walk. It is imperative that these victims exercise as much as they can to keep the blood flowing and to keep their minds as alert as possible. Mama was accustomed to taking a walk to the corner and down the block to the next street but not crossing. I felt comfortable with this until one day she didn't come back. I panicked! She was like a child who had run away. She was really so helpless! All the emotions and thoughts rose to the surface as I envisioned what might have happened to her. Naturally, I began to blame myself, feeling that I should not have let her go alone. I felt others would blame me, and I also knew I could not live with the guilt I would feel if she had been hit by a car. My emotional upheaval was for nothing. She had not gone the path she always took but apparently when she went out the door she turned left and went across the yard and down the creek, quickly becoming lost and confused. When I found her she was as scared as I was. I believe that being unable to envision the way back or the way somewhere is one of the first indications that something is wrong.

From then on, I only let her walk to the corner and back again while I watched from the yard. I also learned the hard way not to take Mama with me to the store and expect her to stay in the car while I ran in for one item. She could not remember that I had told her to stay in the car, nor could she remember that I would be back, so she got out of the car to hunt me. Fortunately, I rushed back out before she had wandered into the main thoroughfare. So what did I do when I had to go to the store? I took her in with me but this was not satisfactory either since she could not remember that things were for sale and not for the taking or eating. I've concluded there are no simple answers to these situations.

Once we went to the grocery together, and when I got back to the station wagon with groceries, I realized that I had locked my keys inside the car. I could see them lying on the seat. I told her I had locked the keys inside and we'd have to go back inside the store so I could call Ted to bring another set of keys. For some reason, this frightened her and I could not get her to sit down where I told her while I made my call. Here I was trying to reach my husband who was not in his office, and she was going out the front door of the store saying, "I'm going home! I'll walk home!" My husband's secretary was trying to locate him, and when she would come back on the line I would be gone trying to retrieve Mama from the parking lot. I was almost on the verge of tears when a young bag boy asked if he could help. I told him my problem and he quietly said, "Ma'am, did you know that the back window of your wagon is down? I could crawl through and open your front doors." What a relief! I felt as if Mama and I both would have been hysterical in a few more minutes. Perhaps my aggravation at myself caused her to feel fear and anxiety. I shudder to think what might have happened to her if she had gotten away from me and walked out into the traffic.

13

Emotions—Ever Changing

Lest I sound as if I carried this load all by myself, let me hasten to say that an incapacitating illness involves and touches every member of the family living in that house and even those members of the extended family. How true that "no man is an island."

We tend to transfer feelings, to make another the object of our frustration, to snap at the ones we love the most, and to let our guard down about every little thing. Of course, everyone has to have a place and a person with whom to do that. But we can easily abuse the privilege if we aren't careful. In the tense pressure of the ever-demanding care of a loved one, we are prone to forget how often we have "let our hair down."

Caring for mentally or physically ill, aging parents can erode a marital relationship very fast. I began to look with envy upon my husband as he carefully shaved, showered, and dressed in a fresh shirt, tie, and suit each morning and left saying, "I don't know when I'll be home, Honey," and here I was stuck here all day feeling sorry for myself thinking, *After all, it's his mother, but I'm the one whose life is changed and disrupted! I am the one answering the same questions all day long and cleaning up messes I didn't make.* I imagined how nice it would be to have a job in the marketplace —to be able to dress up and use perfume, drive my car downtown to a job in an office where everyone could carry on a sensible conversation, where I would go to lunch with the women in some out-of-the-way place or maybe skip lunch and shop for something special on my lunch hour. How nice to be mentally stimulated by the business world with its demands (forgetting how cruel that can be, too).

How easy to think only of ourselves! I tended to fantasize about the "beautiful and intriguing" people who would come to my husband's office that day for counseling. I would wonder if he would notice how nice the women looked and remember the way I looked as I stood in the kitchen that morning mopping up spilled coffee in my "grubbies" with no makeup on. It is amazing how miserable we can make ourselves when we let fatigue, self-pity, or jealousy take over our minds and thoughts. If someone came to the door would he think *she couldn't possibly be the minister's wife*? Frequently, I had to get hold of myself and tell myself over and over how foolish I was to think those silly thoughts.

Several years later after Mama had died, I overheard our third son, Paul, tell a friend, "My mother used to look like a high-school girl 'til Grandma came to live with us." That remark stunned me and stirred emotions I had not felt for a long time. I found I was resenting what I interpreted to be a situation that had stolen my youth and my youthful appearance. I felt a certain pleasure that Paul had said that and at the same time a bit of embarrassment at what I must look like to him now. I know I was uncomfortable with the situation at the time. I have often reflected on it, and I am now sorry I felt that way. It was almost as if I were blaming my "precious" mother-in-law for my getting older. How utterly foolish!

First, I had to remember that I was a creature created in the image of God. I remembered that the Lord is my strength, and whom shall I fear? Again, I read that He never allows us to have more trouble that we can bear. He is faithful. In praying, I would frequently remind the Lord that He knew my frame of dust, because He had made me.

O Lord, thou has searched me and known me.
Thou knowest my downsitting and mine uprising, thou understandest my thought afar off.

Thou compassest my path and my lying down, and art acquaint-
ed with all my ways.

For there is not a word in my tongue, but, lo, O Lord, thou
knowest it altogether.

Thou has beset me behind and before, and laid thine hand upon
me.

Such knowledge is too wonderful for me; it is high, I cannot attain unto it. (Ps. 139:1-6, KJV).

My husband never failed to tell me how much he appreciated
my caring for his father and mother. He would often flatter me by
saying he didn't know another woman anywhere who would do
what I was doing. My ragged emotions needed this kind of balm
and affirmation—I ate it up. Never did he give me reason to think
his devotion for me had cooled. I knew he really loved me completely, and I also knew he didn't need a whining wife to add to his
burden of serving a large church as pastor and doing all the other
things expected of him. Had I forgotten that he too was carrying
the burden of his mother's illness? What did I expect him to do in
the morning? Go out looking like a tramp? or like me? The problem was not with him but with my attitude and emotions. Frankly,
I felt trapped and I was fighting to be freed.

And speaking of being freed—I recall more than once thinking
when things had been especially bad for me. *I wonder just how far
the gas in my car and the money in my purse could take me if I just
got in my car and started driving, telling no one where I was or when
I would be back. Which way would I turn when I reached the top of
the hill? How long before Ted missed me? What would he do, would
he be upset, would he understand? Would he be surprised or even
care? Then, who would they take for granted? Who would clean the
bathrooms, mop the floors, cook the food, do the laundry, or answer
the numberless questions over and over again*? I came to my senses
and realized I couldn't do that to Ted or to Mama. What was
happening to her or to me was not something that had been mali-
ciously planned. It was just something like a risk we take when we
live in this old world. I felt wicked that I had even entertained

such a thought. After all, I needed them as much as they needed me. Since no one else had thrown a pity party for me, I just did it myself. I did agree "for better or for worse" one day many years ago and any way I measured it, it has all been for the better. Few women in this world have had the happiness that I have had in my marriage.

It bothered me that I could no longer keep a spotless house and a beautiful yard. Cleaning house and keeping house has always been a kind of therapy for me. Running the vacuum, immersing myself in the noise of the motor, seeing the floors become clean, the dust disappear from the furniture, and the windows sparkle once again is a sort of cleansing for me. I often pray when I clean. It is a wonderful time for confession and praise. I had enjoyed my role as a homemaker, and I had developed my own little system. Now it was disrupted. I am prone to schedule or time my chores too closely, and then interruptions throw everything out of kilter.

On Mama's better days, when she was more lucid, she wanted to help; and everything I started to do, she would say, "Now I know I could do that!" But she couldn't. If I refused, she seemed hurt. If I let her try, it only delayed me, and, of course, most of the time she couldn't remember how to do it. Once I thought, *Surely she can string beans!* I showed her how, explaining carefully about taking each end off. I thought she had the hang of it, but when I checked on her in a minute or two, she was simply breaking them in half without stringing them. She would want to dust, but she only hit at things and would soon forget what she was supposed to be doing. I know she sincerely wanted to help, but her mind just would not stay stable long enough for her to complete a task. At every turn, as she was following me around, she would say, "Why, are you doing that?" or "What are you going to do now?" Before her disease progressed to this point, she wanted so much to be useful but now she just could not follow through. If I were to say, "Are you going to finish the dusting or would you like me to?" she would probably say, "Did you want me to do that? You should have told me."

I often struggled with the emotions of resentment and pity, and either one brought on guilt. I hated myself when I would resent something she did or said. I would feel guilty when I would wish she weren't there. Once I remember thinking that perhaps God would strike me with Alzheimer's disease for my ugly thoughts. How could I forget that He is a God of love and not vindictiveness? Someone has said that guilt is like pain, it tells us when something is wrong and needs mending. Thank God, we can work through guilt by grace through prayer to achieve peace in our heart.

I hated it when Mama wet the floor or the couch. She did not want to wear protection and waterproof garments; or if she did, she would remove them and I would not know it. I tried to keep her favorite chair or place on the couch covered and protected. Most often accidents would happen when I least expected it. As some people grow older, the muscles get more lax and control is more difficult in this area whether or not they have Alzheimer's disease. What we experienced was more like a child that was not toilet trained. The most successful thing for me was to set the timer on the stove and take her to the bathroom at a given time. We could never trust her to go to the bathroom on her own or to tell us she needed to.

We could not talk without her contributing something totally irrelevant. We could not have friends over; we could not have dinner as usual; we could not leave her alone; we could not take her many places. She couldn't turn things on and off, like the television, because she would pull the knobs off or turn every knob so that we would lose the picture and it would take an expert to straighten it out. She would forget to turn the water off at the sink or lavatory. Living in a two-story house made us fearful she would lose her footing on the stairs.

Once we thought we heard her up in the night and Ted jumped up to see. He started down the stairs and stepped on our Siamese cat Cleo, who was sleeping on the steps. His foot slipped on her slick fur and he flew to the bottom of the stairs landing on his backside, and poor, frightened Cleo flew out over the stair rail into the hall. She screamed that terrible cry that Siamese cats are known for, and headed for the basement where she belonged. Mama was not up but we slept so much on edge that we thought we heard her. Ted hurt his back and poor Cleo had the wits scared out of her. Later, Cleo had a nervous breakdown and had to be put to sleep. (I hope this incident didn't contribute to that.) Neither of us ever really slept soundly. People with Alzheimer's disease don't sleep well either and tend to wander around at night.

Another change that took place in our family life was that our son, Mark, stopped bringing friends by. He seemed to be spending more and more time away from home. This was not like him at all. He is the only child that we possibly could have afforded to send away to college, but he chose to stay at home and go to the University of Kentucky in our city. We were delighted but surprised. Our home now lacked that certain stability he had come to depend on. It was difficult to study; thus, more and more he came home to eat, sleep, shower, and then go out again.

We had two other sons and their wives living in our city, and frankly, I often felt they should have given me some relief now and then but rarely was that the case and never unless I asked. I do understand how daughters-in-law would surely feel no obligation to get involved in this situation. I know they did not realize how pushed to the brink I often felt because one in particular was not hesitant to ask me to baby-sit. I was even accused of never being able to talk of anything else except what a hard time I was having. In other words, people don't want to hear another complain, regardless of how needful a listening ear is. It is easy for outsiders to imagine that the care giver is having to stay at home anyway, perhaps small children would be a diversion. At an earlier time, before Mama and Dad's illnesses, it was not unusual for all our extended family to gather for dinner on Sunday or at night. I would cook and we would enjoy each other. When I became the primary care giver, I couldn't do that so often or not at all and they didn't always understand. It seemed to appear that I was using Mama as an excuse not to have them over. This was not true. In short, as much as family members love each other, they don't always meet the needs of one another. I confess that I was becoming very self-centered and resentful.

The Lord sent a wonderful couple to help us, the Whites. Mama loved them and would cooperate with them. We shall always be grateful for their help. They were not the only ones who shared our burden either. There were some other ladies at the church who would offer to sit and give me a chance to get out now and then. How do people survive without the support of a caring church?

After Mama came to live with us, she joined our church. Her Sunday School class gave me a lovely gift that I enjoyed for several months. They told me someone would meet Mama each Sunday as I brought her in the building and would take her to Sunday School, take her to the rest room, and sit with her in the worship service. Afterward, they would again take her to the rest room and bring her to me after we finished greeting the guests. This was wonderful—I loved them for that!

But even that seemed to bother Mama a little. If she and her care-taker friend for that Sunday sat where they could see me, Mama would look at me with such pitiful eyes, so much as to say, "Why can't I sit with you anymore?" She never mentioned it to me, but her eyes seemed to tell the story. She seemed so glad to get back with us after church. For months, she put on a good front in church. She couldn't carry on a conversation but she was so pleas-ant and smiled when people spoke to her that it was hard to detect she had a problem. It was a long time before many people knew about her illness.

In those days, it seemed I was looking for something to feel guilty about. I knew I was not giving my husband the attention he needed and deserved. I was failing my daughters-in-law and not meeting their needs. I was worth very little to my church and its activities. My prayer life almost degenerated to such self-centered-ness that I found it difficult to pray for others. I had absolutely no civic involvement. I was finding it difficult to maintain an interest in how I looked. I was disappointed in my housekeeping. In addition to all that, I hated myself for feeling guilty because really I knew I was doing the best I could under the circumstances. I resented Ted's accepting so many counseling appointments and letting himself be pulled into so many committee meetings and church activities. After all this was *his* mother.

Why did this have to happen to Mama? She was such a good person and didn't deserve this kind of a break. Why not some wicked, mean person that had no regard for God or His church? I wanted to blame someone for this mess we were in. But whom? Yes, I was tempted to blame God, or at least be pretty "put out" with Him. At the same time I knew the Word said that He sends the rain on the just and the unjust and to live in this old world carries the risk of disease, illness, accident, disappointment, sorrow, and, ultimately, death. One thing was certain: I didn't cause Mama to be stricken with this horrible affliction. But I had to stand with her in it.

"Oh, my Heavenly Father, I plead with You not to let this terrible disease fall on any other members of our family. If this request is not according to your will and one day I am destined to deal with this ailment, then I beg you to make my life short so that I will not heap indignities upon myself and my family.

"Father, I don't want to live in Your beautiful world and not be able to enjoy or comprehend it. I would rather die than not be able to communicate with my friends or family. I don't want them to remember that I was unable to function as a normal human being. Please deliver me from dependency on other people. I want to stay useful and able to do for others as long as I live. I don't mind Your taking me home to be with You but let my family remember me as a contributing member of society and Your kingdom. But Lord, if my request is selfish and my lot should be a debilitating disease, then please give my family the spiritual, supernatural strength they will surely need. Forgive me, Father, for often being less than the best You have planned for me. I love You, Lord."

14

"We Can't Go On Like This!"

It had not been a good day, to say the least! I felt drained, tired, misunderstood, short-tempered, put-upon, angry, and just about any other emotion you want to name including being sick. I was losing weight, and I had the feeling I couldn't go on indefinitely like this. It seemed each day there would be another crisis that would take me further down the path of no return.

At dinner that night Murphy's Law prevailed—if it could happen, it had that day and then repeated itself. We had reached that place of trying to decide what would or could be sacrificed. Already I had begun to realize that it was partly our children and our relationship to them. They didn't come around as often, and we were talking less and less on the phone. It was too easy for misunderstandings to occur. I was edgy and tended to take exceptions to every thing that was said—sometimes reading far more into something than was intended. I had the feeling they were thinking, *Surely Mother, with no small children at home, can handle one old lady; she doesn't work outside the home. Dad does the mowing and helps her at night, plus Mark is still living at home and he can help!*

Later that night there was another bad scene with getting Mama to bed and down for the night. I came back downstairs and Ted was on the phone to his sister, Ruth. I overheard him saying, "If I don't do something soon, I'm going to have two women with mental conditions in the nursing home—my wife and my mother!" None of us had wanted it to come to this. We honestly thought we could manage. Ruth was particularly firm against the alternative of the nursing home. Some months, maybe a year earlier, Mama had been in the hospital. Ted and I had felt that would have been a good time for her to go into the nursing home, but Ruth could not bring herself to do that. It was particularly difficult for her to manage Mama since she was working full time. I could not hear her answer on the other end of the line but I knew Ted was right.

The house was gradually being sacrificed a little at a time as changes were made. When one stepped inside the front door, the whole house smelled like a poor-quality nursing home. Urine smell in carpet just will not come out without professional cleaning, and at the rate we were going I needed to have that done every week.

I felt my role as a pastor's wife had long since been sacrificed. People seemed to know that I did not have time to talk, visit, or counsel over the phone or in person. Now I needed to be the recipient of counsel not the counselor. So many places I would ordinarily have gone with Ted, I had to forego. This was a new experience for me because even when the children were small we either took them with us or we had a sitter. Sometimes we did have a sitter with Mama, but it isn't easy to find sitters to sit with an adult who is ill.

The next day we began to look into the various possibilities in our city. This was no easy task. It did not take long to eliminate most of them when we walked in the door. Finally, we decided on one that was not our first choice in some respects but it was nearby and I knew that would be a factor on a day-to-day basis. The closer she was to us the more often we would see her. We went out to talk to the administrator and to have a tour. I found it interesting that in all of the nursing homes we visited, the front offices, the "living rooms," and the front porches all looked so homey and inviting, but most of the time it is the unseen parts that make a difference in the care given.

Financial consideration had to be given as well as the quality of care. We were trying to find the best we could that satisfied all these needs. We made a choice. Going into a nursing home had not been discussed with Mama so now I had another emotion to deal with. Would she feel that we had rejected her when she needed us most? Or, could she still reason to that extent? How often had I heard her say in years past that she hoped she would never end up in a nursing home. I was experiencing relief and at the same time a feeling of betrayal. I consoled myself somewhat because we were having another problem to deal with. Mama's blood sugar was very high, and I had been unable to get it down with the diet and oral medication. I could not make her understand why she could not have certain foods that we had. She could not understand why we ate ice cream but she could not. Sometimes she would even cry, thinking she had been denied something she enjoyed so much. It was worse than denying a child something. As a result, we found ourselves slipping around eating foods she could not have, But if she caught us, then she was sure we didn't love her anymore or we were just too stingy to share.

The nursing home we chose called and gave us a date to admit Mama. Upon checking the calendar, we found that Ted would have to be out of town for an important meeting on that date. We dared not refuse that date after waiting this long, because we were fearful one would not be offered again for some time. Ted felt terrible about this and offered to cancel his trip, but I felt the Lord was just working this out in His own way. I assured Ted that I would ask our son Jon to help me and we would admit Mama. Mama was always particularly fond of Jon and I knew he could manage her as well as any of us.

Mama was not even aware that I was washing and getting all of her clothes ready and packed. We did not tell her that we were going until the last minute. As fate would have it, that day was one of the best days she had had in months. When Jon came, I told her that we were going to admit her to a small hospital at the edge of town. "Why?" she asked, "I'm not sick!" I told her that I had been unable to get her blood sugar under control, and at this little hospital they would be better able to monitor it and to serve her exactly the kind of food she should have. Of course, she asked, "How long will I be there?" I replied, "I really don't know but we feel this is the best thing for you. I have talked with your doctor and he had made arrangements for you to be admitted this afternoon. Jon will be going with us and help you get settled in." That didn't seem to be much comfort to her as much as she loved him.

When we went for admitting everything seemed fine; she made no significant comments. As we were later going down the hall to her room, she turned to me and said, "This place is full of lunatics! If I stay here long, I'll be crazy as they are!" There are no words to express fully my feelings. My heart was pounding, and I really felt I had betrayed her into the hands of strangers and she was nothing but a little child. Again the thoughts—*Who or what must be sacrificed? How could I have done this to her when I loved her so much?* I felt I had told her a half truth to get her in here and wouldn't you know this was the most lucid day she had had in months? At that moment I felt nature had played a bad trick on both of us. I began to feel that perhaps I had been too emotional and should not have given in to my feelings so often. In other words, did I force my own husband to do this? Was this just to save my own mental health? And now, I had made my own son a party to this! No wonder Ruth had refused earlier to do this—surely this was one of the most difficult things anyone could ever have to do.

Then the thought hit me! *If I were mentally ill or had a dementia of some sort, and she were well, would she be a party to having me committed to a nursing home? Why did I suddenly remember all those times when she cared for me and my babies?* I consoled myself with the thoughts that I did not make this decision independently and it was true that if we did not get her blood sugar down, it would lead to other more serious complications. I told myself also that maybe they could do something for her that we had been unable to do and she could soon return home with us. No wonder she thought the place was filled with "lunatics" when she saw stroke victims tied in wheelchairs begging to get out, or persons jabbering incoherently or grabbing at everyone who passed by. Oh, how I wished she were on that day as she had been for so many days recently—oblivious. She would not even have noticed others if she were.

The room assigned to Mama was on the front where she could see visitors come and go. It was a sunny, pleasant room with a private bath and a large chest of drawers that would amply hold all her belongings.

Her roommate seemed pleasant enough, and it was obvious from the beginning that she had no mental impairment. We thought this would be good and perhaps she would be a challenge to Mama and would be helpful to her as a newcomer. But it didn't work out quite that way. Her roommate was also very possessive and didn't want Mama encroaching one inch over her half of the room. Then, there was the problem that Mama couldn't remember what was hers and what were her roommate's things; hence, Mama was accused of stealing. This blessed mother-in-law of mine, who wouldn't take a crumb of bread that didn't belong to her was now pictured as a thief. How ridiculous! But it happened! We tried to make amends and tried to explain to this other lady that Mama didn't understand or remember what was hers and we'd be glad to replace anything she took or misplaced. I tried to remember her roommate was sick in other ways and basically had no family in town to visit her.

Things grew worse. Finally one day, we were told that they were moving Mama to another room because she had become combative and had hit her roommate. If she continued this way, they would have to restrain her. We couldn't believe this—and still don't! Why, she had never given any indication that she was combative. How we dreaded this for Mama, for by now several months had passed and she could find her way to and from the dining room and the sitting room. If they moved her, it would be like admitting her all over again, but there was nothing we could do. They moved her. From that time on, she went further down-hill at a greater pace.

She was moved into a room with a comatose lady and in a sense had the room all to herself. This meant there was absolutely no stimulation, not even quarreling, which apparently was better than nothing. Once more Mama could not remember which chest of drawers was hers, so often she would have on clothes that weren't hers and much too small. The comatose lady was a small woman.

The room was at the far end of the opposite hall from where she had been. Little traffic came by. The one window looked out on the area between two buildings, so there was little to stimulate her from the outside. One of my friends asked her husband to put a bird house just outside the window so that perhaps as the birds built a nest, Mama would become interested in them. She did not realize it was there. When I would mention it to her and point out that the birds were building a nest, she would seem interested but would soon forget all about the birds.

I made a family collage of pictures, many of earlier years, thinking that would spark some remembrance. I put names under each, but it was obvious the names meant little. I tried to help her identify the family, but it only seemed to confuse her. By now she was having real difficulty remembering any names at all. She often confused Ted with her husband.

Once when Ted went by to visit with her, she met Ted with this message.

"Do you know where Theodore is? He's been gone for hours and I have dinner ready and getting cold. I'm afraid something has happened to him!" Ted replied, "Well, Mother, you know he is a grown man and can take care of himself. If I were you, I'd not worry another minute about him. I am sure he is all right. Why don't we just go ahead and eat while the food is still good?" She said, "You are right, I'm not waiting any longer!"

That seemed to satisfy her and she did not mention Dad again for a long time.

There were many times when she seemed to know family members but couldn't call their names. One of my sons went to visit with me. I said, "Mama, do you know who this is?" She smiled brightly and said, "Well, he's one of 'em." I wish now I had not put her memory to the test. I should have said, "Mama, this is Paul. He is our third son and he has come to visit with you." So many things I wish I could do over—for both of us.

Another time Ted was cutting her toenails and she, realizing I guess, this was a nice thing for him to do, said, "You are the best boy I got!" To which he teasingly replied, "And the worst one, too." She said, "No, you're not—that other one is." Not long after we admitted her to the nursing home, her daughter, Ruth, came to visit. At first she didn't recognize her. When I said, "Mama, this is Ruth," she immediately went into a tirade about where Ruth had been and why she had not called or written. I felt like this took Ruth a little by surprise because Mama had gone down considerably since Ruth had last seen her. This accusation was so unfounded because Ruth and her family wrote often. Mama just could not remember. Most of the time we found her mail unopened. She either couldn't or had forgotten how to open letters.

We know so little about the human mind—even the experts know so little—but it seems that a person with Alzheimer's disease searches unconsciously for identifying persons or objects; something to latch on to. This is why we try to do the same things in the same way so they can identify more easily. After Mama changed rooms at the nursing home, she seemed to gravitate to the nurses' station in the middle of the wing. Many others were there as well. There was a sitting area and some windows that looked out on the golf course. Many of the patients were also rolled in their wheelchairs to this area so the nurses could keep an eye on them.

Mama found a lady about her age who looked for the world like Mama's sister, Grace. She always sat in the same place on the couch, and Mama sat by her. I never heard her friend say a word, but I would frequently see each of them pat the other, or smooth a wrinkle from a skirt. Some times they would just hold hands. Mama seemed so happy with her friend and for months they were almost inseparable except for eating and sleeping.

One day Ted received this frantic phone call from the nursing home asking him to come or at least to talk to his mother because she was hysterical, thinking he had died. He asked to speak to her then, before he went. When he asked her what was the matter she said, "I thought you had died!" When he assured her he was fine, then she said, "It must have been Ruth!" No amount of talking would convince her that they were both fine. He immediately went out to see her. When he arrived he was told by the staff that Mama and her friend had been sitting on the couch as usual and her friend had just dropped her head over on Mama's shoulder. Apparently, that was not an unusual occurrence, except this time her friend had died. Of course, in the midst of getting her friend emergency treatment, Mama was ushered away and all she could piece together was that someone she loved had died and was being taken from her. The staff could not console her so we were called. Ted then called Ruth and let Mama hear her voice. She seemed to believe him then, but for some time she would just begin to cry but couldn't tell us why. We guessed that she missed her friend but could not verbalize her grief to share with us.

Every traumatic thing seemed to push her farther and farther away from reality. She seemed to withdraw more and more, and her unnatural actions seemed to intensify.

She was assigned to a table in the dining room with others, but no one liked to eat with her because she would eat off their plates or do "funny" things. So she ate alone most of the time. I often would try to be there at mealtime and it was heartbreaking to see her trying to eat soup with her hands. I must admit the food was not much of a challenge or thrill, but I am sure it was nourishing. Besides, a diabetic's diet is never too appealing. Residents of the home could be rather unkind, too. If someone got to the wrong table, they were quickly told to move. Alzheimer's victims do not remember which table is theirs. To them one table is as good as the other. They probably don't remember having a table assigned to them. Names are usually on the tables but often they have forgotten or lost their glasses so they can't see the names.

Many churches have a ministry with the residents of nursing

homes. Our church did with the one where Mama lived. One Christmas my sitter/friend went out early and bathed and dressed Mama to come to the Christmas party. Our family was going to be there to sing Christmas carols and the ladies would serve refreshments. When my friend finished and seated Mama at her table in the dining room, she went to help the other ladies with the refreshments. Mama disappeared and when we found her she had gone back to her room and put on two or three pairs of slacks under her skirt. It was time to start, so we brought her back and had our program.

On impulse, Ted said, "Mother, come up here and sing with me!" She immediately got up and waltzed up to the piano. They sang not a Christmas song but "In the Garden." She sang every word of that song in her beautiful clear alto voice, never missing a word or a note. It was beautiful—we all wept. Five minutes later she didn't even know what she had done. We were all astonished that she could remember the words and music. From our experience, it seemed that her musical memory was the last to go.

It would appear that the very present is the only thing real to a person with this type of dementia. Mama always seemed glad to see me, but often when I would offer to take her for a ride she refused. We frequently brought her home for a meal or for holidays, but even at Christmastime she seemed uninterested in what was going on around here. Sometimes before the meal was over, she would say, "Well, I guess I'd better be getting home." She would repeat this often and now and then even seemed to get anxious when we didn't hurry.

Apparently, she did not ever remember living with us. At that time we lived at the foot of a hill. As we would head down the hill and into the driveway, she would say, "Who lives here?" or "What are we stopping here for?" Often I would ask if she remembered living here and she would say no or not answer me.

We found that summer picnics outside were a good time for us to have her with us. The grandchildren seemed to fascinate her, and there was plenty of room for them to romp and play. She loved watching this. We did not have to worry about spilled things or her incontinence. However, even enough of this was enough and she would begin talking "going home." Sometimes this made me sad, but, on the other hand, I was glad that she felt she had a home with familiar surroundings.

I could find many things to be unhappy about with the nursing home. I felt the one we chose first surely did not get better but rather went down. The stench was terrible when one walked into the wing where the patients lived. I felt they hired just about anyone who would do that kind of work. Of course, they had a registered nurse on duty most of the time, but I saw people sitting wet too long and personally experienced some things with Mama that were very disturbing to me.

Once we had to make a trip, and I let the home do her laundry. It looked terrible. Colors were washed with whites, underwear ruined in too hot a dryer, and on and on. Things were lost and never recovered. She definitely was not bathed often enough. I always bathed her as did two of my friends who visited her regularly. From what I was told, the home only bathes them every other day or less. She had a private bathroom, but she could not bathe herself anymore nor could I get her out of the tub by myself. I would have to call for help and often wait for them to come. She was frequently found in her own excrement. Once my friend found her lying on her bed with no clothes on and the door wide open. Her teeth were never cleaned unless we cleaned them. I helped her clean them for as long as she could coordinate her hands. For some reason that I can't explain, I found cleaning her dentures the most difficult thing I had to do for her.

It was obvious that the nursing home was not getting better, so we began a search for another one. The reluctance we had in doing this was knowing that it would be so hard on her to learn everything again. This would be the third time since she left our home that she would have to learn where to eat, sleep, and sit. We were successful in relocating her and it proved a good thing. Even though it was strange, the attitude of the staff seemed different and she seemed brighter and more responsive. She seemed to smile more and her appetite was better. I often went to have lunch with her, and she even got back to the place where she would try to introduce me to her new friends. She couldn't get names out so I helped her by introducing myself and telling them that I was her daughter-in-law and that she was like a mother to me. Once she was in such good spirits that she tried to be funny. One of the waitresses in the dining room was grossly overweight and after she passed by Mama said, "Boy, she looks like she stayed at the table too long, doesn't she?" Then she laughed and laughed. Of course, I joined her and told her if I didn't stop eating lunch with her so often, I was going to be the same way. We enjoyed that light moment together—but it didn't last long. I never cease to be amazed at the mind of an Alzheimer's victim, how alert and rational they can be one minute and the next be lost in their own little dark world.

Ted and I both felt good about the arrangement at the new facility. The administrator was a beautiful Christian, and the home was church-owned. Finding the right place for your loved one is so important. At best, it is perhaps the most difficult thing a child has to do regarding his parent. Maybe we make it harder on ourselves than we should because of the feelings of guilt we carry, believing our parent thinks we have rejected him or her. I am confident this would be more true where the parent has all of his or her mental faculties functioning properly.

The months dragged on and our lives took on a little more normalcy which included frequent trips to the nursing home. We all knew this was the best arrangement for both our family and Ruth's, but I suppose we never felt completely good about it. It was exceedingly difficult to realize that this childlike creature was once the strong woman we had known.

In the predawn hours one Sunday morning in early February, the nursing home called to say they were admitting Mama to the hospital with irregular heartbeat. Ted said, "Shall I meet you there?" but the administrator knowing it was Sunday and Ted had to preach in just a few hours said she did not think it necessary, that this was just a precautionary measure. She suggested that he go on over to the hospital after morning worship. This we did and found Mama resting quite comfortably. Many months earlier, Ted had instructed the doctor and hospital that no heroic measures were to be employed to resuscitate Mama. We knew she had no quality life to look forward to on earth and to extend this hazy, unreal existence for her would be unthinkable.

I must say again how unpredictable the human mind is even when it is ill. When we got to the hospital, Mama seemed so normal and lucid. She looked at Ted and said, "Son, there is something bad wrong with me!" Of course, she was being monitored and watched closely. We stayed with her that afternoon and she talked with us as she had not done in some time. She remarked how much she liked the colorful blouse I was wearing and asked about the family. When we had to go, we told her we would be back right after evening worship, before going home.

There was a fellowship time after church at which we felt we must put in an appearance and while there we received the message, "Ted, your mother has just had a heart attack and died!" As Ted stood there dry-eyed yet broken, he said ". . . Absent from the body, . . . present with the Lord. Blessed be the name of the Lord!"

On the way to the hospital Ted remarked to me, "We didn't lose Mother tonight, we lost her years ago. This woman that we have cared for and loved was not the woman I have known for so much of my life as my mother. As I look back over the years, I realize that she died a little every day." As we arrived at the hospital, there waiting for us was our beloved physician who had struggled with us all these years. It is rare to see a Christian physician, a deacon, and friend who makes himself available to share a moment of grief as this man did. The three of us stood around Mama's bed and wept, not for her but for ourselves as we thought of our loss in what might have been, has she not been ill with this dementia.

We learned from Dad's passing that the funeral should be where the friends are who have stood with you. So we had the funeral in Lexington with Ted conducting it. It was difficult for him to do, but I think he always regretted not conducting his father's funeral. How appropriate that the son they raised and dedicated to the Lord, whom they faithfully prayed for, the one in whom they took such pride and pleasure, should be the one to give the eulogy and to commit Mama's earthly house back to the dust from which it had come. So a few days later we again gathered at the old Zebulon Cemetery in Toccoa to inter Mama next to Dad under the shade of the old cedar tree. Oh, but their lives haven't ended! The truths and precepts they instilled in their children live on and in their grandchildren, all of whom can "rise up and call her blessed."

> Who can find a virtuous woman? For her price is far above rubies.
> The heart of her husband doth safely trust in her so that he shall have no need of spoil!
> She will do him good and not evil all the days of her life.
> She seeketh wool, and flax, and worketh willingly with her hands.
> She is like the merchants' ships; she bringeth her food from afar.
> She riseth also while it is yet night, and giveth meat to her household, and a portion to her maidens.
> She considereth a field, and buyeth it; with the fruit of her hands she planteth a vineyard.
> She girdeth her loins with strength, and strengtheneth her arms.
> She perceiveth that her merchandise is good; her candle goeth not out by night.
> She layeth her hands to the spindle and her hands hold the distaff.
> She stretcheth out her hand to the poor; yea, she reacheth forth her hands to the needy.
> She is not afraid of the snow for her household: for all her household are clothed with scarlet.
> She maketh herself coverings of tapestry; her clothing is silk and purple.

Her husband is known in the gates, when he sitteth among the elders of the land.

She maketh fine linen and selleth it; and delivereth girdles unto the merchant.

Strength and honor are her clothing; and she shall rejoice in time to come.

She openeth her mouth with wisdom; and in her tongue is the law of kindness.

She looketh well to the ways of her household, and eateth not the bread of idleness,

Her children arise up and call her blessed; her husband also, and he praiseth her.

Many daughters have done virtuously, but thou excellest them all.

Favor is deceitful and beauty is vain; but a woman that feareth the Lord, she shall be praised.

Give her of the fruit of her hands; and let her own works praise her in the gates (Prov. 31:10-31, KJV).

My friend, Mildred Wade, an author, has shared with me "A Letter to My Mother."[1] With her permission I share it verbatim.

Dear Mother,

As far back as memory serves me, I have enjoyed our visits together. We have made castles in the sand, mixed batter for cakes, rehearsed my lines for school plays, shared feelings, ideas, and friends, watched each phase of my children's growth, and prayed together. Through it all—insignificant events and highlights—our visits together provided time for us to talk. And our talks are one of the things I cherish most.

With you in a nursing home now, I am no less eager to visit, but I find myself at a disadvantage because I don't know what to expect. When I visit next week will I be Aunt Hattie, Mother? Or your school chum listening to whispered secrets? Or your mother tying a red ribbon in your thick black hair, now thin and gray?

At times I am all of these, and more. I respond not as your daughter, but according to your recognition. It's like the game we played when I was a child. I was the Little Colonel, shaking my short hair as if it were long curls. You leaned back to look at me objectively and declared I was much prettier than the Little Colonel could ever be. You shed a tear at my Joan of Arc speech. Your applause was enthusiastic as I became, in turn, each character in *Little Women*. And you laughed delightedly as I recited "Giuseppi de barber is greata for mash; he's gotta de bigga de black mustache, good clothes and good styla and plenta good cash." We both knew when the pretense and games were over.

Now you have introduced new games, Mother, and they are not pretense. They are confused reality for you, and sad frustration for me because I don't know the unwritten script that can change minute by minute.

Several weeks ago the cloudy veil covering your mind lifted as I sat facing you, trying to respond to your questions as I thought Aunt Hattie would have. But she died when I was a baby and I didn't know her. It hurt me to see the distress I was causing you when I couldn't, as Aunt Hattie, recall the name of your nearest neighbors, and didn't know about Uncle Oscar's rheumatism, and could not describe the dress I gave you for your tenth birthday.

Suddenly your eyes glowed with recognition. You grasped my shoulders and exclaimed, "You're not Aunt Hattie! You're my daughter! My own daughter!" You hugged me tightly and said my name over and over. I sensed that you knew your mind had been wandering in darkness and had suddenly encountered brilliant sunlight. My mind kept repeating, "You're back, Mother. Hang on! Hang on!" We embraced long enough for me to blink away the tears I didn't want you to see. Then your voice rippled with laughter. I was delighted and laughed, too. You took your arms away from me and, looking at me lovingly, you smiled and said, "It's so good to see you, Aunt Hattie. Thank you for coming."

No, you don't know me sometimes, Mother, and you are no longer the mother I've always known. Our roles have changed. I am now the mother; you are the child. You seem content with your new role; mine is uncomfortable. And sometimes my feelings about you are uncomfortable.

At my last visit you recognized me instantly. "You look tired," you said, getting up from your comfortable chair and insisting that I sit there and relax. Once again you were my mother, and I was your child. You sang hymns softly and I watched you, remembering many other times you met my needs.

When I left later I said I'd see you soon. But I wanted to tell you that although a stranger inhabits your mind much of the time now, and you don't always know who I am, I know that my presence stirs pleasant memories within you, and we will have many more visits together, Mother, you and I.

Your devoted daughter,

Mildred Wade

Part III:

These Things We Have in Common

15

"Now About Old Age . . ."

"Youth is the gift of nature, but age is a work of art."
—Garson Kanin

In the Old Testament, it seems that old age was an eagerly anticipated happening. By our standards Moses was an old man when
he obeyed God's call to go to Egypt and demanded of Pharaoh
that the children of Israel be freed to go worship their God in the
desert. Old age was revered and people had respect for their elders
and sought them out for advice and wisdom. God even promised a
long life to his children who honored and respected their parents.
He also made promises to the patriarchs about the continuation of
their line in their old age. It appeared to be a goal to achieve.

Not so today! The society in which we live has elevated the age
of youth to unbelievable heights. The success of yuppies is herald-
ed as the goal to strive for. There seems to be an unwritten law
which says that if you haven't made it by the time you are forty,
forget it—you will never make it. You may even be considered a
failure by some. Truly, this is the age of the twenties and thirties!

Advertising is bent toward the youthful or at least toward those
who are anxious about retaining their youthful appearance. It is
almost impossible to see or hear advertising for skin care or weight
control without being reminded of how important it is to remain
young in our thinking and control our weight so we will look
young whether we are or not. I surely agree that weight control is
important for our health, regardless of our age. However, youth is
touted to be a state of utopia—nothing else matters so long as we
stay slim and youthful looking. Unfortunately, we have all been
indoctrinated with this until we have come to agree with it in our

own minds. I find myself thinking and even saying to my husband, "I don't mind getting older so much as I dread looking old!"

Have you ever seen a commercial on television for eye makeup for the mature or wrinkled woman? No, and you probably won't! Has anyone ever dared to advertise truthfully how nice it is to have a "potty tummy" or "saddlebag legs"? No, they won't do that either. Ideally, we "gals" want to remain unwrinkled, clear-skinned, flat-tummied, full-bosomed, muscles taut, slim, and clear-eyed. The "guys" want to remain tanned, muscular, big-chested and flat-bellied. It is a fact of life—that is our ideal. Instead, one morning we wake up to body changes. Taunt skin has become double skin under our chin, our backside seems to be slipping down around our knees, and our slim waist has suddenly developed a spare tire. What hangs from our upper arms we refuse to claim as ours. Long-sleeved garments become more attractive to us all the time. Looking down our arms to our hands, we realize we not only need a face lift, we need a "hand lift." Somebody said we may fool others about our age for awhile but our hands are a dead giveaway.

Is that really a dowager's hump developing? Oh, oh, oh, she should have taken her hormones more faithfully! Most of us really don't want to get older but the alternative is not too attractive either.

There is a distinct turning point in our lives regarding age. Remember how anxious you were to become sixteen so you could get a driver's license? or single date? Certain things were not allowed either by parents or the law until we got to be a certain age. When that happened, we felt we had literally arrived. Nothing could surpass that wonderful feeling!

My grandson David, who is now thirteen asked me, "Ginny, do you know I am now an adolescent?" (Do we ever!)

"Yes, I know that, David. How do you feel about it?"

His reply was a classic honest answer. He said, "Well, some days I like feeling as if I am becoming a man, but other days I want to be a little boy and maybe stay that way. Do you understand what I am saying, Ginny? It seems that everybody wants me to act like a man and are saying so, but I still feel like a boy most of the time."

I am probably guilty of being one of the "everybodys" who is pushing him toward manhood. As adults we are not consistent. We do want children to take on more responsibility, stop doing childish things, or saying "dumb" stuff. When they tell us, however, how many years or months it is before they can drive the car, we panic and begin putting on the brakes.

This attitude of "Isn't it great to be getting older?" prevails until about the mid-twenties. Then we began consciously or unconsciously trying to reverse the aging process. I remember thinking that if I didn't get married before I was twenty-five, I probably never would have an opportunity. I wanted to make sure I wasn't left out in the cold, so when Ted proposed at eighteen I said yes and married him at nineteen.

Now that I have my own set of crow's feet around my eyes and smile lines have taken up residence on my face, I am amused and sometimes nearly smug about seeing or hearing my daughters-in-law bemoan the fact that they have a wrinkle "about" to come. We all fall into the trap of supporting a multi-billion-dollar business to buy all sorts of reported remedies to retard the aging process. I lead the pack--so this is not a criticism but an observation. You know what many women would like for Christmas next year? A face lift! Since most of us can't get it, we resort to mud packs, egg yolks, vitamin creams, and a long list of products that are supposed to help us look younger. We undergo scrapes, peels, burns, and lot of other things one doesn't usually associate with the face, in order to look a little younger.

But, alas! nature and time win again! It is a losing battle, but we still need to do all we can to outdistance them. Shall I be really honest? I think I would love to stay young all the days of my life, but that presents a problem when one has grown children and adolescent grandchildren. "Vanity of vanities, . . . all is vanity," so says Ecclesiastes 12:8.

My handsome father-in-law fell into that trap. . It was a common sight to see him take out his knife or tweezers and either cut off or pull out the gray hairs in his mustache or on his hands. He would comment to us about his approaching old age. At times he acted as if he wanted to be an old man, but his actions belied his words.

People are funny creatures. Some deny getting older by continuing to dress as teenagers or by wearing whatever is "in," such as mini-skirts. Some are blessed with a baby face or a slim figure and can get by with this pretense a long time. All too often people, men and women, will have affairs as if to prove their virility, youth, or attractiveness. Some will even admit they wondered about their attractiveness to the opposite sex and, when the opportunity presented itself, refused to think of the sordid consequences that more often than not accompany sexual sin. Spouses are devastated and families split apart.

People fail to realize that rejection of a spouse or anyone is the severest of emotions and growing older is a welcome scene beside that. Isn't it interesting that many people are reluctant to tell their age if they are past thirty-five, until they get to be ninety or more, then they want it told and even announced on national television? Try getting people to promote into an older group at church. Honest people sometime resort to lying and some even quit coming, rather than tell their age.

Shortly after we came to our present pastorate, an elderly lady died whom my husband did not know very well. At the wake he asked the surviving sister how old the deceased was. She looked around to see who might be listening and said, "Well, Preacher, I'll tell you, but if she knew I did, it'd kill her!"

Age doesn't seem the most important thing when we are young and so much in love. It doesn't seem to bother a girl if she is three or four years older than the man, but wait until she hits fifty. Wild horses couldn't pull that admission from her. When Theodore and Lena Sisk were married, they "adjusted" their ages on the marriage license so that she was only two years older than he, rather than four. He advanced his a year and she lowered hers a year. Perhaps the fact that he was a teenager and she in her early twenties prompted them to do that. We would have been none the wiser except for Mama's sister, Aunt Grace, who had all the births of the Smith family recorded in the family Bible. I doubt that birth certificates were issued or births recorded at the county courthouses in those days. We might say, "What difference does it make?" Well, it made a great deal of difference to Mama all her life.

Have you ever noticed how some people seem to feel free to ask people whose hair is gray if they are retired or when they are going to retire? This question may threaten job security in the mind of the employee and the employer. We have come to think that when a person reaches his or her sixty-fifth birthday, they are ready to retire. Even churches are conditioned to this thinking. Most churches seeking a pastor will not even consider a man past fifty, unless he is particularly outstanding. Rather, they want a man who is in his thirties or forties with years of experience and wisdom. Those creatures are rare. Just because a person has reached sixty-five doesn't mean that he is ready to quit. I feel that this generation of young people is having a hard time coming to grips with the fact that most people who have reached the retirement age of sixty-five still have years of experience and wisdom to offer their professions. Too often they are put on the sideline in favor of younger people.

The fact that large corporations are urging their older employees to take early retirement rather than lay off younger people encourages that kind of thinking. They seem to want to retain the creativity of the younger people. Many companies are giving handsome retirement packages to employees who will retire early. Some of these people are only in their fifties. What will they do? Some don't want the responsibility of trying a new business venture. Learning new technology and ways is more than they want to tackle after being with a company for twenty-five or thirty years. I know some of these people personally, and they are bored to death. The very things they looked forward to are now becoming a bore. After all, how many days a week does a person want to play golf or fish? A man in good health and a right attitude will soon get the jobs his wife has planned for him around the house done and then feel as if he is under foot or in his wife's way. Often the retirement package does not allow for extensive travel, so that isn't an option. I have concluded that what makes persons feel and act young is knowing they are needed and are making a significant contribution on behalf of others. Feeling useless and unneeded makes a person think, *Well, maybe I am getting old,* or *I guess I have lost my enthusiasm for life or my job* or whatever the responsibility might be.

Age is a relative thing. One is not necessarily as young or as old as one's chronological age would indicate. Physical or mental indicators of aging are varied and do not necessarily keep pace with chronological age. Life is full of milestones or events that mark passages of life for most of us. As I stated earlier in this book, my mother-in-law taught me many things, not the least of which was her philosophy of life.

She told me that when she and Dad were married she thought surely no two had ever been so in love—that life just didn't get any better or more wonderful than this. She had someone to love just her in this particular way and just for herself. Then, the children came along—admittedly earlier than they had planned or expected; but after all, weren't the children a visible expression of their invisible love? It was all right and somehow they would manage. They did, with the help of the Sisk grandparents who shared most of the expenses.

It seemed that hardly any time had passed, before the children were ready to start to school and another phase of life started. School involvement with PTA and being a homeroom mother was a new adventure. The ability to take the kids along with them wherever they went was another plus. It was wonderful! Once more, she had the day to herself after the children left in the morning to walk to school. They came home for lunch so she could see them at midday, but she still had some independence and time. Then came high school and graduation. Where had the years gone? Within two years both children were away in college and another era dawned.

The empty-nest syndrome set in for awhile but soon that passed as they looked forward to the times when the kids came home for weekends and special events. This was great—almost like when they were just married and were just two. As the years slipped by, there were weddings of children and then grandchildren came along, and this was the best time yet according to her. Thus, her philosophy was that every phase of life is the best. I think she is right. No longer do I wish my life away as I did before I was sixteen years old.

We can all agree that we do not wish to grow old, but we know that we can do nothing to prevent it, except die and that is a poor alternative. Growing older in this day is surely not like it was a hundred years ago or less. No longer are those over sixty-five put on a shelf, unless that is their choice. There are numerous organizations and agencies working to see that they have as good an old age as possible.

Communication keeps older Americans in touch with their families even though they live far away. By means of telephone, more elderly are able to remain in their own homes longer because they can be almost instantly in contact with their doctor, dentist, friends, church, or even account executive at the brokerage house. Many communities have a "lifeline" so that the elderly can just press a button and be connected to immediate help should they fall or suddenly need help. Some organizations can arrange for persons who live alone to be called each day to see if they are all right.

Television is truly a window on the world and people don't have to feel cut off from the rest of civilization, even if living alone.

Transportation is more affordable and frequent than ever before. Guided tours around the world and across the continent are everyday things and offer a wonderful opportunity to meet people with similar interests. For some people, it is a chance of a lifetime to travel just about anywhere their heart desires with someone to tell them exactly what to do. Someone will take care of every detail, including registering them at the hotel and getting their bags to the room. For the groups that Ted and I have led, we even took care of passports and airline tickets once we were airborne and all arrangements made. That way no one could inadvertently pack them in luggage that was long gone. Instructions were given as to what to take, what not to take, where we would go, what time to get up, when the bus left for sightseeing, even when we would eat, or at least what the options were. We have dispensed medicine, mended suitcases, given instructions for calling home, and counted bags and people until we did it in our sleep later at home. Lasting friendships have been formed from these tours.

Being among the elderly these days is a different story. The graying of America is a force to be reckoned with politically. Many lobbying organizations on the state and national levels are working for the senior citizens. Seniors need to be in touch with those who are working for them and not be hesitant to contact them.

Senior-citizens centers have sprung up all over the nation and they offer a variety of services from classes of various sorts to daycare for the elderly. The American Association of Retired Persons has a representative who will assist in filing Medicare/Medicaid forms and will help with income-tax preparation.

One lady in my church who is an employed senior herself tells me she needs an assistant to help her in the job placement office she operates from the senior-citizens center in our city. She cannot find enough people to fill the requests she has for seniors to work in the various capacities available. This gives seniors extra income, contact with the public, a feeling of being useful, plus the opportunity of sharing their wonderful cache of experience and wisdom. People of this age can stay active and useful if they are physically and mentally capable.

Another lady in my church works every day in the dress department of a thriving downtown department store where she has been employed for years and years. She walks a mile to and from her apartment every day, rain or shine. She has the slim figure to show for it, too. She is eighty-eight and retirement is not part of her future plans.

Another woman who is also eighty-eight demoted herself to a younger department in Sunday School last fall because she didn't feel a part of "that old women's class" where she belongs agewise. One is not necessarily as old or as young as one's chronological age would indicate.

John Wood, writing in *Modern Maturity*, tells of a seventy-five year-old man who was being discharged after a stay in the hospital. Concerned, the hospital staff inquired about who would care for him during his convalescence. "Don't worry," he said, "Mom will take care of me." The staff laughed, thinking him a witty character. The next day, a ninety-two-year-old woman hobbled in and took her son home.[1]

The aging process has been receiving the public's attention through media and legislation and other concerned groups, but too often the focus is on such dysfunctional aspects of aging—as poverty and disease, and is usually discussed in derogatory terms. Understanding what the aging process is really all about will enable us more clearly to understand those persons who are aging around us. Jean Maxwell (*Centers for Older People*, New York: The National Council on the Aging, 1962) has suggested that persons recognize ten basic concepts of aging. These are generalized statements that provide a foundation for studying the aging process.

1. Aging is universal. It is common to every population and is not just a modern-day scandal in Western civilization.

2. Aging is normal. "Growing up" is spoken of with respect; "growing old" with fear. This fear develops from the stereotyped picture of aging as a loss of faculties, beauty, energies, and memory.

3. Aging is variable. Each individual ages in a unique way.

The state of a person's later life develops from a former personal life pattern.

4. Dying is normal and inevitable. It is difficult for many to accept the idea that while a full, satisfying life is being lived, death can be anticipated as a meaningful closure of life.

5. Aging and illness are not necessarily coincidental. Again the stereotype image lingers; but individuals should prepare for healthy old age through improved living habits in early and middle years.

6. Older people (those over sixty-five) usually represent three generations. In no other life stage is such a wide age span lumped into one group which may include parents, grandparents and great-grandparents.

7. Older people can and do learn. The capacity to learn new things and relearn the old is not necessarily diminished by old age. Learning patterns may change from youth and the speed of learning may slow down, but the ability to learn appears to be culturally determined, not restricted by years.

8. Older people can and do change. As one grows older many readjustments become necessary. Mates die, housing situations change, new activities are developed, and new friendships established.

9. Older people want to remain self-directing. "They never want to decide anything for themselves" is a common complaint concerning older people. But such dependency is learned, usually as a direct result of loss of purpose and self-respect. To prevent this loss when an older person undergoes a change in life, his self-direction should be maintained as much as possible. Even if an individual cannot enjoy complete control, one must have a feeling of having contributed to the decision-making process.

10. Older people are vital human beings. While physical disability is often associated with mental inadequacy, it should be recognized that the need for physical help in crossing the street does not mean that the person does not know where he is going.

When one can appreciate that each older person is a living, interesting human being with whom association can be rewarding, and beneficial, then a positive interaction can be anticipated, regardless of the width of the generation gap.[2]

I have surmised from this research that old can be defined in a number of ways. It appears that "young-old" is from sixty-five to seventy-four, "median or moderate old" is seventy-five to eighty-four, and "old-old" is eighty-five and over. Aren't we all anxious to be or to remain, one of the "young-old?" In order to do that we must think young, act young, and talk young.

First of all, take good care of yourself physically. Often people who live alone do not eat healthily. If you don't know what is good for you (whether you are a man or a woman), read information on the subject and find out. The library is full of good books on nutrition, or the bookstore will sell you an arm load of books and magazines about how, what, when, or where to eat. Your doctor, whom you should see regularly, will recommend cookbooks on how to eat if you have a heart condition or diabetes. So what if it's not how you learned to cook! You can learn a new recipe. Even people who live alone and hate the thoughts of cooking should learn how to eat correctly, avoiding fats, high cholesterol, empty calories, and high-sodium foods, whether they eat at home or in a restaurant. Learning to cook correctly and inviting friends who are also alone to share meals and expenses is a good idea. Even men who may have never learned to cook nor given much thought to eating correctly can learn how to eat correctly and to cook if they have any inclination for cooking.

Our appetites may be geared to the time when we did more strenuous work or were more active around our homes, but we must be aware that as we grow older, we need fewer calories. These should include good wholesome nutrients that our bodies need. Consuming fewer calories doesn't mean we need fewer vitamins and minerals. This means we need a well-balanced diet.

Avoid the temptation to snack on sweets or junk food just to satisfy the hunger. Sometimes an older person's appetite decreases especially following an illness so that he or she may forget to eat or doesn't feel that it is worth the effort. In most cities, older people may take advantage of the "Meals-on-Wheels" program or something similar. In a rural area, perhaps arrangement could be made with a neighbor to share dinner with you, even delivered, for a fee. Some of the senior-citizens centers offer a lunch program. The telephone directory or the local newspaper will probably give an idea of what is available. Call the Department of Human Resources in your area or ask your telephone operator to put you in touch with the agency that can help you.

Good health doesn't consist of just eating healthily but also exercising. Most seniors are not too turned on by areobics as most folk generally think of aerobics. It is most important that you check with your physician about an exercise program. Exercise is important for your physical, mental, and emotional health. You may start out simply by walking around the block twice a day or doing the usual housework you have always done as part of your daily living pattern. Once you get permission from your doctor, think about what you would like to do for exercise. Well, yes, golf is good exercise if you walk and pull your bag on a cart, but how often do you do that? Effective exercise needs to be something that you do every day, or at least three times a week.

Walking is an inexpensive and most effective exercise and can be done by more people safely than any other exercise. To walk in the open air and see the beauty of God's good earth is invigorating. It makes you realize how great He is and how insignificant we are. In winter when the weather is very cold or bad, join the multitudes who do mall walking early in the morning. People with arthritis are usually told to keep moving. Most people by age sixty-five have some arthritis. People with heart disease need to keep walking, too, especially if a doctor has recommended it. It is a proven fact that walking helps keep blood pressure under control, plus it is an aid to weight loss.

Of course, there are other good forms of exercise. If you have been a member of a health club or the "Y" for years and are in the habit of going there regularly, you should continue if the doctor says it is all right. Swimming is great exercise and also good for arthritis. There are terrific low-impact water exercises that many people are enjoying. If you don't have arthritis in your hands, bowling is fun exercise. There are other exercise programs for seniors at a health club, the "Y," and many churches. Many corporations now have built-in facilities for employees to exercise on their lunch hours or after work. Avail yourself of every opportunity to exercise. Take the stairs, not the elevator, unless stairs are forbidden by a physician. Continue to mow your yard, do your own housework, garden, raise flowers and vegetables, and do the odd jobs you have always done around the house for as long as you can. You are adding days and maybe years to your life. All the above is, in my judgment, part of acting young. The more active we are, the younger we feel.

But what about thinking young? The more birthdays we have, the more people feel at liberty to ask our age, or to talk about age. They seem to want us to feel and think old. Let's not allow ourselves to be caught in that trap. Continue to read what is going on in the world, try to learn something new each year, such as how to use the computer, play tennis, paint, or sew. Why not take a foreign-language class, a real-estate course, or any number of things in order to learn something new? In other words, be willing to take on a challenge and believe you can do it. Unless you have a disease like Alzheimer's or some other mentally debilitating illness, you can. Refuse to think that your life is about over and you'll just coast into glory from where you are now. Think of all the years of experience and wisdom you have stored up and how much help you could be to the younger generation. Who knows, perhaps a few would even listen to you? The experiences God has given you could be used for His glory if you are willing. Offer to teach a class in your church Sunday School or even work with the babies in the nursery once a quarter. The more involved you are in good things, rewarding things, the younger you are going to be and feel. Maybe you have never had the time to do volunteer work but now you do. Hospitals, as well as many other good organizations, need men and women to be volunteers. Volunteering is not just for the women. It is very consoling for a male patient to see a male volunteer when he is admitted in the hospital. The contact with people is exhilarating and you have the feeling of being able to contribute. The amount of time given is up to the individual.

Do things with your grandchildren. Go to their soccer games, to the school play, or to their recitals. Offer to chaperone a school activity. Try to learn to understand some of the lingo they use and don't appear too shocked at the way they dress or act. Remember they are trying to establish their own identity and feel they must appear "cool" to their peers. (Are we so different?)

Do something you have been putting off doing all your life! Don't feel you are too old! If your health is good or even reasonably good, go ahead and fly to Hawaii or to Alaska. Drive through New England in the fall or whatever you have talked about and planned on but somehow never felt you could do . Even if your spouse is in the beginning stages of a crippling disease either mentally or physically, don't wait any longer. It will be wonderful to reflect on, when the road gets rough later on. It will be something to recall that you both enjoyed doing together. These days travel can be as expensive as you want, but it is also possible to travel at reasonable costs. Look into all the possibilities and choose something you can afford and will enjoy. Take a compatible couple along with you to share expenses and experiences.

Be careful how you talk, or you will appear to be "old-old" and then you will feel old. Go easy on sharing "how it was when I was growing up" or else or it will be a dead giveaway how old you really are. Don't feel you have to contribute your ideas or experiences to every conversation that you overhear. Wait until you are asked or it seems appropriate. People who live alone tend to talk too much or clam up and say nothing. If you have lots of time to talk on the telephone, remember the person you are calling may not have that much time. Always ask if the person can talk at that time and remember it is better to call more often than talk too long at a time. If you like to talk on the telephone, ask your church to give you the names of some shut-ins who would welcome a chance to talk. Children and old people have been accused of having no real concept of time, and there is a lot of truth in this. Keep well read so you have something to talk about besides the past and your aches and pains. Write down some of the fantastic or unbelievable stories from your past and preserve them for your grandchildren. When they are older, they will be delighted to have this memento from your past. It will make them feel a part of their heritage.

In order to be one of the "young-old," take stock of what you need to do or continue doing as you go into this exciting time of your life. Take stock of what you are now doing that you shouldn't, such as smoking or drinking or other bad habits. You say you can't change now? That is one indication of old age—resignation that change cannot take place. Are you a couch potato? Get up and begin some exercise, even if it is just stretching and walking through your house or yard. Turn off the television and spend some time in God's Word and world, asking the Lord to help you accomplish this task of taking care of the temple of the Holy Spirit—your body.

Set some goals for yourself for the next five years. Be realistic and don't try to accomplish everything at once. For instance, if you need to lose weight, learn how to eat more healthily and read up on the nutrition facts. Maybe you could begin by leaving off sweets or fried foods, switching from regular to low-calorie type dressings. It is a fact that the harder we make it on ourselves, the more likely we will be to cast the challenge aside and go back to our old habits.

Act, walk, think, and even dress young (don't go overboard on this last one), and listen for people to comment that you certainly don't seem as old as you say you are. And now a private word to the "gals." We don't have to look old because we can "color rinse" our hair when the grey starts appearing; we can watch our weight so that "close to" our marriage weight is a reality all the days of our lives; and we can keep our mouths closed about how old we are (unless we have a husband who loves to tell how old he is and in the next breath tell everyone you are the same age as he). Seriously, we owe it to ourselves, our spouses, our children, our friends, and our Lord to act, think, and be as young as we can because our bodies became the temple of the Holy Spirit when we first believed.

Are you dreading those retirement years when you and your spouse will be home all the time? Do you imagine that life will come to a screeching halt and all the things you once loved to do together will no longer be fun or enticing? Sure, there are some changes ahead, but retirement years may be the richest days of your life. What about all the things you have wanted to do but didn't have time? Remember the books on the best-seller list that you wanted to read but didn't have time? Well, now you have. Your local library is a wonderful place to find all kinds of great reading materials and usually great surroundings. Put a sandwich in your pocket and take off on a cold rainy day to spend the day at the library or your favorite bookstore. In our city, we have a bookstore that provides a crib and playpen for children, hot coffee and cold drinks for browsers who want to spend the day. Recently, I noticed a pianist was playing soft classical music for those who were browsing. I honestly look forward to taking advantage of that. In addition, most libraries sponsor activities including lectures and movies.

It is a healthy mind that continues to thirst for knowledge, and it is also a sign of a young mind. Have you noticed how many median and older adults are returning to college? Some are entering institutions of higher learning for the first time. Adults are serious students. They know the value of money and they have a reason for going with a goal in mind. Colleges are delighted to have these older students. They help the financial crunch most colleges are feeling right now in a time when the enrollment of younger students may be decreasing. Some of these older students are returning to finish a degree or to prepare themselves for a new career; some were unable to go to college when they finished high school; and still others return to pick up something they missed when they were undergraduates. Many of the colleges and universities offer a variety of courses for credit and noncredit. If school is the fulfillment you have been looking for—go for it!

Not to be overlooked are the changing sexual lives of the elderly. Here again, another freedom for the older couple—sex without fear of pregnancy means it can be relaxed and enjoyed. While not all older partners still find pleasure in sexual intercourse, age knows no bounds for enjoying the pleasure of touching that comes with warm, close contacts. An interesting observation of the surviving population of older women is that they experience healthier emotional well-being when they have access to intimate, affectionate relationships.

From our childhood we have had ingrained in our minds how wonderful and thrilling it is to be a youth or to be youthful. Then, at the time in our lives when we are faced with all the physical, mental, career or professional changes, we are also faced with some of the most traumatic happenings or events in our entire life. For instance, birth, death, marriage, divorce, and remarriage all have a significant effect at any age. They affect the elderly more critically, especially those who are in their mid-seventies or beyond. Events such as the death of a spouse, the loss of friends, or changes in environment are harder to take in these later years. Often when a spouse dies, the surviving partner is not included in activities with the couples as they once were. He or she seems more often than not to be invited only when a hostess needs to round out a number at her dinner table. Often the widowed spouse feels funny, as if someone is trying to play Cupid and is therefore, hesitant to accept the invitation. If it is declined, it is often not extended again.

Other threats that may occur after the death of a spouse are the fear of reduced income, loneliness, isolation, dependency, or immobility. All of these often result in depression. Remember how we planned for our children's education and all the other good things we wanted them to experience? We must also plan for our own growing old. Many people avoid the discussion of death, insurance, estate planning, and other things usually associated with growing old, but we must accept the challenge of making plans for ourselves and include our children or the person who will be responsible for our well-being when we are unable to do it ourselves. Ruth Kay, the editor of *Plain Talk Series*, in consultation with the National Institute of Mental Health says it is never too early to ask ourselves the following questions:

—What living arrangements and life-style will offer me the best in comfort, convenience, independence, and companionship at a price I can afford?

—What work and recreational activities should I pursue to keep me physically and mentally fit?

—What organizations provide services for the aging that I should know about?

—What medical/health services and benefits, including Medicare /Medicaid, will be available to me?

—What will my retirement income be, together with retirement benefits such as Social Security?

In old age as well as other stages of life, we should accept the challenge as part of life and plan positively for it.[3]

A new kind of problem facing our country today is what to do with this older generation that is living longer and healthier than ever before. A generation or so ago when a parent was left or when both parents became infirmed, they moved in with one of their many children and were cared for as long as they lived. At that time a nursing home was not an option. Today medical science has discovered cures for many of the things that once claimed the lives of older people. What to do with them then was not so much of a problem because they didn't live that long.

The fastest-growing group in our population is those over sixty-five. In 1988, they numbered 30.4 million, or 12.4 percent of the U.S. population. In the decades of the 1970s and 1980s, the over-sixty-five population grew by 56 percent while the under-sixty-five only increased 19 percent. The older population itself is getting older. In 1988 the sixty-five to seventy-four age group (17.9 million) was eight times larger than in 1900, but the seventy-five to eighty-four group (9.5 million) was twelve times larger and the eighty-five plus group (2.9 million) was twenty-three times larger. No wonder we talk about the graying of America.

Some experts have made conservative estimates indicating that by the year 2050, 50 percent of the American population will survive their eighty-fifth birthday. In that year, they estimate that the over-eighty-five population will number approximately fifteen million.

Here in the United States, elderly women now outnumber men by three to two. This difference by sex is even more striking in the upper-age range. In 1984, there were eighty-four men between sixty-five and sixty-nine for every 100 women in that same age bracket. In the eight-five and older population, there were only forty men for every 100 women.[4] On the average, women live longer than men, and as a result more frequently end up living alone. I have been told that if a couple is the same age, the averages indicate that the woman will be a widow for seven years. This fact has a major impact upon their health-care provisions.

Life expectancy has also changed during the past seventy years. A child born in 1900 could expect to live an average of 47.3 years, but a baby born in 1988 has a life expectancy of 74.9 years.[5] Today's sixty-five-year olds can expect to live to an average age of eighty-two.[6] It is predicted that by the turn of the century these expectancy figures will be even higher. This increase is due largely to a decrease in the infant and young-adult mortality rate. Since 1970 the increase has been due to a decrease in the mortality rate among the middle-aged and the elderly.

There are some unique features within the changing demography of the elderly. The Veterans Administration health-care system is facing severe stress as large numbers of veterans age. It is predicted that by the end of the century two thirds of our elderly males will be veterans.

According to the American Association of Retired Persons in their pamphlet, "A Profile of Older Americans, 1989," older men were nearly twice as likely to be married as older women in 1988. Half of all older women in 1988 were widows and there were five times as many widows as widowers.[7]

The majority of older noninstitutionalized persons lived in a family setting in 1988, but the population decreased with age. About 13 percent were not living with a spouse but were living with children, siblings, or other relatives. An additional 647,000 lived with nonrelatives but not in an institution. About 30 percent of noninstitutionalized older persons lived alone in 1988. They represented 41 percent of older women and 16 percent of older men.[8]

On the average, persons over sixty-five visit a doctor six times for every five times by the general population. They are hospitalized twice as often as the younger adults, stay twice as long, and use twice as many prescription drugs. Health-care utilization is greatest in the last year of life.

Attitude makes all the difference in the world, whether one is nine or ninety. The way we view things sets our disposition, our energy level, and our general outlook on life. Recently, I read the article "Aging Upward: How to Win While Growing Old" by Royal H. Roussel in *Aging: Special Issue on Independence*, a publication from the U. S. Department of Health and Human Services.

Roussel at eighty-three has an outlook I envy. He and his wife Dorothy live in a retirement community and are the coeditors of the community newsletter.

Roussel says we should recognize that all of us are aging by the minute and we should spend more time preparing for being old instead of trying to hang on to being young. He further states that life, happiness, and accomplishment are not the exclusive possessions of the young. He notes that he speaks with authority since he has been old for such a long time.

His opinion is that age can be a wonderful experience—a priceless gift. We should see it as a natural development and not as an affliction. He insists that, much to the surprise of most folk, age does not always multiply or intensify miseries and we should accept it as a friend and not fear it as an enemy. He reminds us that aging is the only way we and our loved ones can enjoy a long life—and who can be critical of that? Old age is not a time to retreat from life but to advance in a new direction. We need not creep timidly into old age, he says, but enter boldly, as participants. As one manufacturer advertises, "We are not giving up, we are moving on."

Another new thought came from this clever writer. Roussel says, "Many of the articles about old people that I read have a critical fault. They are written by people who are not old. The writers can see 'old' from the outside only, as spectators and not as participants. They are not yet playing in the game. Often they perpetuate the mythic stereotypes of old people.

"No one is likely to say that growing old is easy and fun. As we age we are often in danger of feeling like stragglers from life, aware predominantly of the burdens and afflictions of our years. Then we are prone to ignore the opportunities that are before us. At this point some of us succumb to miserable oldness. But others fight the psychological and, when possible, the physical effects of aging—and succeed in winning some of the battles." He said, "I chose to fight!"

Roussel has suggested four essential considerations in his timely article on aging. These I'll summarize.

First, it is necessary to keep a good balance between physical and mental capabilities. Neither should be stressful but stimulating; they should complement each other and be enjoyed.

Second, we should know when to back off or disengage. Realize we cannot do everything we once did. We must abandon some of our habits, activities, and interests of younger days while adopting new ones more in keeping with our age—but ones just as rewarding.

Next, it is essential that we be satisfied with life, a condition which can be enhanced by evaluating ourselves carefully as aging individuals and then setting goals that we can expect to attain. As we grow older we have increasing needs for the exhilaration of achievement. Failures cause age to weigh upon us more heavily. As often as possible we must feel like winners—satisfied with ourselves.

In the fourth place, we must maximize our use of time. No one who isn't old can possibly understand how precious time is, what another day of life means, what a blessing it is. Never waste a day or an hour. Enjoy every minute. This is the spirit in which old persons must live. Actually, we should be the happiest of all people. We are blessed with the precious gift of extended life. Who could ask for more?

We lose our youthful appearance; we experience emotional changes; and we encounter variations in our mental capabilities. We can, however, still age upward by gaining wisdom, patience, and understanding. Though our bodies and sensory systems caution us repeatedly of physical and biological changes, usually losses, we find that we have greater inner strength and staying power than ever before.

The social structure of our lives alters in response to new conditions, but we are not dismayed. We accept and enjoy the new conditions as a time of discovery, adventure, and opportunity.

We "see" life differently, but it is upbeat, interesting, and promising. It must be a cheerful outlook, so says Roussel.

Living with oldness is not all bad, not all downhill. We must analyze carefully and then act to compensate for the losses and burdens that advancing age imposes upon us. The goal: grow old under optimum conditions. Age upward!

Roussel reminds us that we as well as the aged live visibly on the very edge of eternity and that death is at everyone's elbow constantly. Only the vulnerability of the younger ones is not so visible.

"In our oldness there is no future. Our past is beyond recall. We have nothing left but the present. It is frightening to contemplate the fact that we have lived to the very edge of the last brief period of our existence. This factor of immediacy can give our life an exciting quality. In these final years, I find that everything is in sharper focus. I 'see' more clearly, 'hear' better, understand more fully, enjoy more completely. All life contracts. Everything is intensified, presses closer, impacts more strongly. Living becomes a beautiful, wonderful experience: above and beyond anything we could know in our earlier years."

We all need a reason to live, something to give life meaning. Goals can provide meaning, something to tie to so that we don't drift meaninglessly into senility. Each individual must list his or her own goals for aging. Roussel says that independence is at the top of his list. He insists that we do not have to become more dependent as we age. He asserts that he is more independent at eighty-three than he was at sixty-three because he has learned how to be old and happy. "I have paid my dues," he says.

"Our minds are marvelous instruments and not thinking will age us faster than just about anything. Your mind wants to work for you. Never deny it that opportunity. Think . . . Think . . . and Think. Innovate, create—we must use our minds.

"I do not envy the young. On the contrary I feel sorry for them. They have so much to learn, so many bumps to experience, so many disappointments to overcome. We old ones are far ahead. I am proud of my oldness and of that which it represents. I am a winner, not a loser.

"Physical fitness is a 'must.' Never give up. I exercise every day with a group of both sexes. It's inspirational. All of us are old. Some have suffered illnesses that have left them partially disabled so that they must go through the exercise while seated. But they are courageous, and they participate in physical fitness. Old people refuse to be defeated. Life is a series of battles.

"Before I go to sleep each night I take a few minutes to analyze my life during that day. Happily in this process I see myself winning many small victories.

"In our oldness we must learn to recognize every victory, to know when we have won and have reason to be proud. If we can win small victories often enough we will realize in due time that we have won a large and very important one . . . that we are Aging Upward."[9]

I am indebted to Royal H. Roussel for his views and insight on the advancing years, especially since most of the things written today deal with the more negative aspects of growing old. He says, "Being old offers an opportunity to find out what really is important."

Beyond these practical views and insights of Mr. Roossel, we in the fold of Christ have the promise of eternal life from the God who cannot lie (Titus 1:2).

Did not Robert Browning say it well in the very beginning of *Rabbi Ben Ezra*?

Grow old along with me!
The best is yet to be,
The last of life,
for which the first was made:
Our times are in his hand
Who saith "A whole I planned,
Youth shows but half; trust God:
see all, nor be afraid!"[10]

16

Dementia

Webster's Ninth New Collegiate Dictionary defines dementia as, "a condition of deteriorated mentality." Dementia is not a disease but a group of symptoms that characterize certain diseases and conditions. For years we seemed to lump all mental conditions of the aging into one pile and called them senility. We know now that this is not the case at all. From reading the dictionary definition of "senile" or "senility," we could infer that senility is a condition occurring at a certain age, regardless. Now we know that is not true. Dementia can be further defined as the inability of the mind to function normally as in thinking, reasoning, and remembering. When it is sufficiently severe, dementia interferes with a person's daily and usual functioning, such as work, social activities, or learning abilities. Perhaps later behavior, personality, or mood swings may indicate that he has a dementia of some sort.

The most common form of dementia today is recognized to be Alzheimer's disease. In booklets produced by the Alzheimer's Disease and Related Disorders Association, Incorporated, we find that some of the more well-known diseases that produce dementia include Alzheimer's disease, Huntington's disease, multi-infarct dementia (strokes), Parkinson's disease, Pick's disease, Creutzfeldt-Jakob disease, Lou Gehrig's disease, and multiple sclerosis. Other conditions which can cause dementia or mimic dementia include hydrocephalus, depression, brain tumors, thyroid disorders, nutritional deficiencies, alcoholism, infections such as meningitis, syphilis, AIDS, head injuries, and drug reactions. Some of these conditions may be treatable or reversible.

Alzheimer's disease is a progressive, age-related, brain disease that impairs thinking and behavior. It is now the fourth leading cause of death among older Americans, according to the Alzheimer's Association. It was first described by a German physician, Alois Alzheimer in 1907 when it was considered a rare disorder. This neurologist-psychiatrist discovered curious tangled fibers in the brains of senile patients. These tangles, called "Alzheimer's baskets," enclosed masses of dead brain cells. Since then, doctors have learned that, as the tangles multiply, more and more circuits are disabled until the tiny "batteries" that store and transmit information can't relay it. Without the involuntary function of these cells, the victim is confused and helpless. The resulting sensation is much like what the rest of us may feel just before falling asleep or immediately after awakening. For the Alzheimer victim, that state continues for hours and eventually becomes irreversible.[1] I recently heard a physician who deals with this dementia every day say that there are more than four million Alzheimer victims in the United States alone. Besides the trauma of a family seeing a loved one deteriorate mentally and physically, the medical and health-care expenses are estimated to cost American families nearly forty billion dollars annually.

The gradual onset of this disease progresses so slowly that most of the time we consider the situation to be age or the natural occurrence of losing a few things or mislaying items. Which one of us has not done that very thing? But the Alzheimer victim may soon began to experience a definite change in personality, behavior, or impaired judgment. He may no longer be able to work with figures, solve problems, use words, reasoning, or judgment correctly. A little later he may have difficulty finishing a sentence or finding the right word; he may start to say something but in the middle of the sentence begin a totally new thought. A person who has always taken great pride in his appearance may suddenly lose interest even to the point of refusing to bathe or shave. For some, this may take a long time for these changes to occur, but for others it may be to that stage before they can admit that something may be wrong.

Unfortunately, an absolute diagnosis can be made only by autopsy when brain cells are examined. At autopsy, Alzheimer's diseased brains show the presence of tangles of fibers (neurofibrillary tangles) and clusters of degenerating nerve endings (neuritic plaques) in areas of the brain that are important for memory and intellectual functions.

Another characteristic of Alzheimer's disease is the reduced production of certain brain chemicals, especially acetylcholine and somatostatin. These chemicals are necessary for normal communication between nerve cells.[2]

The Alzheimer's Association tells us that less than 1 percent of people age sixty-five or younger are affected. However, the disease is present in an estimated 25 percent of those age eighty-five or older. But it can occur much younger as well. The youngest documented case is that of a twenty-eight year-old person.[3]

No one knows what causes Alzheimer's disease. Scientists are continuing to search for a cause and their search is pointing in several directions.

For one form of the disease, called Familial or Uncommon Alzheimer's disease, there is strong evidence that a defect exists in a single gene on chromosome 21, and was linked to a form of Alzheimer's disease that attacks a person before age sixty-five.[4]

But for most patients the genetic involvement is less clear. Although there does seem to be a genetic predisposition for the disease, other factors influence whether or not an individual develops Alzheimer's disease.

As recently as May 8, 1990, the *Lexington* (Ky.) *Herald-Leader* reported on a study by Dr. Allen D. Roses of the Duke University Medical Center in Durham, North Carolina. This study has found evidence for the approximate location of a second defective gene that helps cause Alzheimer's disease, a possible step toward developing a therapy. The gene appears linked to a form of the disease that runs in families and strikes at average age of sixty-nine.

Roses said, "We think that anything we find in what is recognized as late-onset familial Alzheimer's disease will certainly have applicability, or can be tested for applicability, to those people who appear to be sporadic [cases].

"So that if in fact we can find a gene and we can develop a rational therapy based on what we find, that therapy certainly ought to be tried in the sporadic [cases].

"The study was aimed at finding a location for the second gene among the 23 pairs of chromosomes found in most cells of the body. Results suggest a 'very high likelihood' that a defective gene conferring susceptibility to late-onset familial Alzheimer's resides in a portion of the chromosome numbered 19."[5]

Scientists are still exploring the possibility of a slow virus, environmental toxins, such as aluminum, and other physical conditions of an individual that may interact with the genetic defect.

Is Alzheimer's disease fatal? Probably not, although the disease is associated with a shortened life span. The slow, progressive nature of the disease often means the patient will live several years after the diagnosis. It eventually leaves the patient physically less resistant to infections, such as pneumonia which could prove fatal. Since this disease generally affects older people who may be subject to chronic illnesses, this may often be the cause of death.

Can we prevent the onset of Alzheimer's disease? No, it seems that the best we can do is to try to keep the older person in generally good health. If the disease strikes, then we need to help the victim continue to do as many things and as often as he can so that he can remain independent as long as possible. Most of us feel that strides are being made in this area of research, but it is a long, tedious task. Special support and care should be given not only to the patient but also to the primary caregiver. The frightening truth about this nearly-epidemic affliction is that it's a slow, mind-destroying killer that can turn a beloved spouse or parent into a difficult, even troublesome stranger. This disease is surely not selective in its victims.

Multi-Infarct Dementia, or vascular dementia, is mental deterioration caused by multiple strokes (infarcts) in the brain. The onset of MID may be relatively sudden as many strokes can occur before symptoms appear. These strokes may damage areas of the brain responsible for a specific function, such as calculations, speech, or motor skills, and there may be more generalized symptoms, such as disorientation, confusion, and behavioral changes.

Brain-scanning techniques are used to identify brain damage from strokes. MID progresses in downhill steps with periods of stability and possibly some slight improvement in between.

A history of high blood pressure, vascular disease, diabetes, or previous strokes have been identified as risk factors. MID is not reversible or curable but recognition of an underlying condition (for example, high blood pressure) often leads to a specific treatment that may halt the progression of the disease.

Parkinson's Disease patients lack the substance dopamine, which is involved in control of muscle activity by the nervous system. Tremor, stiffness, and slowness are characteristic features of Parkinson's disease. Speech may be slow and movement may be difficult to initiate. Late in the course of the disease, some patients develop dementia. Some Parkinson patients develop Alzheimer's and some Alzheimer patients develop Parkinson symptoms. Parkinson drugs can improve the motor symptoms, but they do not improve the mental changes that occur. In fact, Parkinson's disease serves as a model for drug research on Alzheimer's.

Huntington's disease is a hereditary disorder that usually begins in mid-life and is characterized by irregular involuntary movement of the limbs or facial muscles and intellectual decline. Psychiatric problems are common, with depression and memory disturbances occurring in early stages. The pattern of memory impairment differs from that seen in Alzheimer's disease. As the disease progresses, movements become severe and uncontrollable; mental capacity may deteriorate to dementia. The family history of the disease, recognition of typical movement disorders, and CAT brain scanning provide evidence for a diagnosis of Huntington's disease. A genetic marker linked to the Huntington gene has been identified on chromosome 4. Researchers are working on locating the gene itself. The movement disorders and psychiatric symptoms seen in Huntington's disease can be controlled by drugs; however, no treatment is available to stop the progression of the disease.

Creutzfeldt-Jakob disease is a rare fatal brain disease caused by a transmissible infectious agent, possibly a virus. Failing memory, changes in behavior, and a lack of coordination are some of the symptoms observed in the early stages of the disease. It progresses rapidly, usually causing death within one year of diagnosis. Examination of brain tissue reveals distinct changes unlike those seen in Alzheimer's disease. No treatment is currently available to stop this disease.

Pick's disease is a rare brain disease which closely resembles Alzheimer's and is usually difficult clinically to diagnose. Disturbances in personality, behavior, and orientation may precede and initially be more severe than memory defects. Like Alzheimer's disease, a definitive diagnosis is usually obtained by an autopsy.

Normal pressure hydrocephalus is an uncommon disorder that consists of difficulty in walking, dementia, and urinary incontinence. An obstruction in the normal flow of the spinal fluid causes the fluid to build up. Presently the most useful diagnostic tool is the MRI scan. Possible contributing factors are a history of meningitis, encephalitis, and head injury. In addition to treatment of the underlying cause, the condition may be corrected by a neurosurgical procedure (shunt), to divert fluid outside the brain.

Depression is a psychiatric disorder marked by sadness, inactivity, difficulty in thinking and concentration, feelings of hopelessness, and sometimes suicidal tendencies. Many severely depressed patients will have some mental deficits including poor concentration and attention. When dementia and depression are present together, intellectual deterioration may be exaggerated. Depression, whether present alone or in combination with dementia, can be reversed with proper treatment.

Depression sometimes has the symptoms of the onset of organic brain disease (such as Alzheimer's or other types of senility) and are incorrectly diagnosed as such. It is believe that many general practitioners are not sufficiently trained in geriatrics to pick up on indications of emotional problems; therefore, many patients are treated for physical rather than emotional problems. It is also easy to assume that patients with symptoms of Alzheimer's have the disease and that diagnosis becomes a catchall for any cognitive impairment. Often depressed elderly people have many physical complaints as well as signs of mental deterioration. It is easy, therefore, to label a chronic complainer a hypochrondriac and not take too seriously all his or her aches and pains.

(The foregoing information relating to the various dementias has been taken directly from the ADRDA pamphlet "Alzheimer's Disease and Related Disorders, A description of the dementias." Written permission from the ADRDA has been granted.)

Incorrect medication from multiple prescribers or poor nutrition may also produce false symptoms of organic brain disease, as well as producing body chemistry imbalances and infections. Old age itself is not disabling but the diseases which often occur may be. Much research is presently being done so that correct diagnoses may be made and the quality of life improved for people in their old age.

With all these debilitating diseases that have been reviewed, it is important to try to determine at what stage the patient is at present. How much assistance the patient requires will be determined by the extent of his impairment. For him to make the best use of his remaining abilities, it is essential for his well-being and for the well-being of the caretaker family, to determine early what he can still do. It will help him to retain his feeling of self-worth. Even people with dementing illnesses can retain a little dignity and self-esteem when they are able to do a little something for themselves and perhaps for others.

Some experienced caregivers have suggested as therapy, such things as sweeping the walk, folding clothes, drying dishes, dusting, raking leaves, or simple tasks that might be assigned in which the patient cannot harm himself. As the disease advances, be prepared for uncompleted tasks or ones which have to be done again. But at least it fills the time for the patient and gives him a feeling of having contributed something—it can give his life meaning. Ask the patient to wash his hands and set the table for dinner—so what if the plates and silverware are not in the right place! This simple task can occupy the patient while a meal is being prepared and perhaps aid in relaxing an otherwise stressful situation in which the patient might continually ask the same question over and over.

While scientists work over their test tubes and microscopes, making notes on first one experiment and then another, hoping to find a sure cure and a preventive medicine for these various forms of dementia, there have been some unusual findings to report. The significance of these is yet to be proven.

Insight magazine, March 27, 1989, contained the article "Nose May Be First Site of Alzheimer's" by Dina Van Pelt. I quote from the article: "Nasal tissue found to contain the same abnormal nerve fibers as those found in brains afflicted by Alzheimer's disease suggests that certain changes in the nasal cavity specific to Alzheimer's could allow researchers to follow the disease's course more closely and possibly enable earlier diagnosis. Loss of smell is believed to be one of the first signs of Alzheimer's, and researchers hypothesize that the nose may be the first area the disease affects, possibly serving as the entry point for the toxins, pathogens, or environmental factors that may contribute to the disease. Researchers compared samples of nasal nerve tissue taken during autopsies on nine Alzheimer's patients with autopsy tissue from 14 persons of similar age who had no evidence of the disease. All but one of the Alzheimer samples contained significant amounts of certain abnormal proteins within the nerve fibers, while only two of the nondiseased tissue samples did. The proteins identified are characteristic of brain tissue in Alzheimer's patients and are found in brain cells.

". . . researchers . . . hope to analyze living nasal tissue and determine whether the disease is expressed early on there."[6]

As recently as May 4, 1990, what appears to be a significant breakthrough for dementia-afflicted victims made the national news and was reported in the *Lexington* (Ky.) *Herald-Leader.* It was entitled "Brain Tissue Grows in Laboratory Dish." It was reported: "Brain tissue from a child has been nurtured into a colony of living cells that eventually may be used to replace damaged brain cells of those who suffer from Alzheimer's disease, stroke or head injury.

"Dr. Solomon Snyder of Johns Hopkins School of Medicine in Baltimore said his research team had, for the first time, developed a continuous culture of human brain cells that divide and grow in laboratory dishes. Scientists have long been hampered in their study of the brain because human brain cells won't reproduce."[7]

Having had the experience with an Alzheimer's victim that we have had, I believe I can honestly say that this disease is worse than death—it is living death as one stands by and watches one's family member die a little each day. It is devastating to caregivers to see these once vivacious, strong, loving family members be reduced to little more than contrary children, or silent scared little animals who can't remember anyone or anything. When a person has a disease like cancer, there is hope for a cure. If that is not the case and the person becomes terminal, at least there is an end in sight—with some degree of dignity. Families know how to prepare for that kind of demise, and future plans can be considered for the surviving family. The patient usually has opportunity to "set his house in order." It is the kind of death we know how to deal with, but not Alzheimer's—the death that lingers on and on.

A lot of research has been conducted, and those of us who are familiar with the disease are grateful and continually look for new rays of hope. I am disappointed that government money for research seems to have become a political football in Washington. It seems that militant-type groups who are clamoring for causes like AIDS research are making more headway than other interested defendants of diseases which take more live each year than AIDS-- diseases like Alzheimer's, cancer, and heart disease.

If you or a family member is suspected of having a dementia of any sort, a diagnostic workup by a physician experienced in the diagnosis of dementing disorders should be scheduled immediately. This testing probably will include a psychological evaluation and exhaustive laboratory testing. By doing this, the patient may receive treatment for treatable or reversible conditions. If it is not reversible, the patient and the family together need to begin planning for his future care while the patient is still able to have some input. By ruling out certain things doctors can be fairly accurate from the beginning if the patient has Alzheimer's.

When the patient goes for the results of the tests and to hear the doctor's diagnosis, make sure that he or she does not go alone. Have family members there to reassure as well as to hear correctly what the doctor says and prescribes as a course of treatment. Assuming that this workup has been done in the early stages with the patient still lucid and only having brief periods of memory lapse or other symptoms, she needs to hear what the doctor says so that she can have some input into the plans that must be made. It is important that a mentally healthy person hear the report of the physician because the patient will not remember all that was said and will be confused, repeatedly asking questions. The caregiver can give assurances and correct information if she has been there. Conceivably, hearing the diagnosis could cause the patient to get worse, at least temporarily. This should be a time of tenderness and reassurance; but be sure you do not make promises that you will be unable to keep in the future. Talk to the doctor privately to find out what you can do now to relieve some of the tension and disappointment. More detailed suggestions are made in the caregiving chapter of this book about legal procedures.

One thing that can be done early on is leaving notes posted in conspicuous places in the house, such as when to take medicine, make sure oven is off, and lock doors at night. Leave a note on the bathroom mirror, listing in order how to groom herself and a place to check it off. These would perhaps begin with: take a shower, use deodorant, brush teeth, comb hair, and use hair spray. A note from the caregiver listing how to put on makeup in the proper stages would be helpful. Leave a note on the refrigerator about the food inside and when to eat it. The sense of smell diminishes with Alzheimer's, and sometimes people will eat food that is spoiled, causing many unnecessary problems. Often these people will forget to eat or can't remember if they have. Their knowledge of nutrition is often gone so they eat only what tastes good, like sweets. Try to bear in mind that the victim is just that—a victim, not "crazy," "goofy," or any other derogatory term we might be tempted to use. Try to remember that it is a mind illness, just as respectable and unavoidable as if it were heart disease. This situation is hard for families to accept since our culture demands that we admire acceptable behavior even in children, much less adults. *The 36-Hour Day* by Peter V. Rabins and Nancy L. Mace tells us that "a frequent characteristic of a dementing illness is that personality and social skills appear nearly intact while memory and the ability to learn are being lost."[8]

Maintain your own sense of humor, if possible. Some of the things the impaired one says are really funny and when you laugh with them you are not laughing at them. I have heard from my mother-in-law some expressions I had never even thought about and I might say to her, "Where did you hear that?" or, "I've never thought of expressing it that way!" She may realize then that she pulled a "funny" and we would both enjoy it. If it should turn out to be something vulgar, ignore it or pass it off as simply as possible. I believe it is good therapy for family members to continue to talk to the individual (and not about her in her presence), even if the conversation and answers don't make sense. At this point, a smile and a hug are good for all concerned.

Sometimes it is hard to remember that the impaired person still has a great need for affection. Maybe that need is one of the last things to go. Just as touching and loving are very important to an infant, so it is with older people. A pat, a hug, a kiss on the forehead, an arm around the shoulders, or any other means of good taste affection is reassuring. This type of tangible caring is important and needed by normal older people more than anything else—it is especially true of the mentally impaired. Haven't you ever noticed how affectionate retarded children are? They literally cling to the one showing affection and interest.

One caregiver expressed shock and indignation at some crude things her father who had been a pastor said when he became afflicted with Alzheimer's. She was amazed that these words and expressions would even be in his vocabulary. Perhaps this is a good place to say that just because the Lord has saved us doesn't mean that He took away our awareness of sinful nature. Ministers hear lots of things they don't want to repeat or to make part of their speech patterns. When the mind is affected, these things sometimes come out.

Personalities change and gentle and genteel persons who have never cursed or displayed a bent for violence, may suddenly become combative, hard to handle, and even dangerous, making close supervision a must. Violence often makes a family realize that institutionalized care is the only option left for them because of other family members in the home who might be harmed.

Frequently in the beginning stages of a mental disorder the patient may appear to have become just ornery and hateful, uncooperative and spiteful, as he accuses a spouse or other family members of taking things, refuses to take a bath, or to speak to a familiar neighbor. This kind of behavior can be very hurtful to a devoted spouse or child who is caring for him. Demented persons often seem to have become experts at starting arguments and in general trying to be disagreeable. Once family members know the loved one is sick, it is easier to cope. It is hard to do in the latter stages of a dementia but we must remember that we are dealing with a person with feelings. He may not be able to express them, or unwilling to try, but he is still a human being, one we have loved. I remember very vividly my husband saying of his mother, "This woman is not my mother; we lost mother years ago." That was true but even that shell of a person represents the person she once was.

When dealing with excited or angry patients, try to keep your voice down, remain calm and reassuring; remind them that you love them and that you wouldn't do those things you have been accused of. Don't confront but rather distract. Say, "Would you like a cup of tea with me?" Don't say: "That isn't true"; "Try harder, you can do it"; or "Don't ask me that again!" It may help you to remember that they are probably afraid and are trying to prove to themselves as well as to you that they are still in control, though obviously they aren't.[9]

Needless to say, when a mentally impaired person moves into your home, it will necessitate changes. Once he is there, try to establish a simple routine that you can follow from day to day, such as meals, baths, or exercise. Don't change furniture around; keep him sitting at the same place at the table. Keep things simple, tidy, and uncluttered. Keep noise at a minimum and have as few people around as possible. Sometimes taking a demented person into an extra large room or hall adds to his confusion and disorientation. Avoid conflicting stimuli, such as having the television and radio on at the same time, or children playing loudly in the same room with the TV. Try to get him to rest twice a day. If time permits, the caregiver should rest at the same time because of the sleep lost at night. You may have to make adjustments in your home, such as picking up rugs that the patient might fall over, putting a gate at the top of stairs, installing bathtub grab bars, taking knobs off the range when not in use, unplugging the TV, keeping sharp knives hidden, and any number of other things that the patient seems to find that we never would have thought of.

To those of us who have normal mental faculties it is bewildering why those with dementia can't follow through on the instructions written out, when we know they can still read. What most of us don't realize is that though they can read they forget the first part of the message before they have even read the last part. It is the same way with a spoken message. We tell her we are going to a neighbor's house to borrow the morning paper. We ask if she understands; she assures us she does. But before we get to the neighbor's, she has forgotten. All she knows is that when she looked around we were not there and she was frightened. Caregivers become a security blanket, a rope that will lead them out of this terrible maze and darkness. Many feel if they could just get home again, out to their car, or where their spouse is, everything would be all right. We can understand a simple message so easily; we wonder why they can't.

My mother-in-law loved the soap operas in the afternoon, but after awhile they meant nothing to her because she could not remember the characters or what had gone on before in the plot. At this stage television only added to her inability to cope.

There are many other bizarre behaviors that we see in people with dementia. There is wandering or getting lost, inability to sleep and keeping the rest of the family up, refusing to use proper eating utensils, eating makeup, trying to open the car door when the car is moving (thank goodness for seat belts), masturbation or fondling the genital area, improper use of hands in the bathroom, giving money away (if they have access to some), crazy clothes combinations or no clothes, and on and on. There is really no way that one caregiver can prepare another for all that could happen. One can surely understand after being a caregiver why Mace and Rabins called their wonderful book, *The 36-Hour Day*, because the days seem endless but the energy is over soon. I consider this

book must reading for those going through this ordeal or antici-
pating doing so any time in the future. I regret that I was not
aware of the book, though it came out too late for part of our
experiences.

The poignant story I am about to relate had special meaning for
me as a minister's wife. This is the only life I have known as an
adult because I knew when I married that my husband would be a
pastor. I have known the joys, the sorrows, the highs, and the
lows. I have learned to weep with those that weep and rejoice with
those that rejoice.

This is the story of Bob and Betty Davis as told to Tom Watson,
Jr. and printed in *Christian Herald*, October, 1988.

Bob had served as pastor of the Old Cutler Presbyterian Church
in Miami for fourteen years and had led them to grow from a
handful to a congregation of over 2,400. He seemed to thrive on
such a challenge as this, and the future looked bright for this fifty-
two-year-old former All-American, who had once been offered a
chance to play with the Chicago Bears. His wife Betty was a vital
part of his ministry.

For some time, Bob had been having difficulty organizing his
notes in sermon preparation. He couldn't remember Scriptures
that were familiar to him. He couldn't read and concentrate any
more. He couldn't balance the bank statement. And his sermons
were having less and less theological "meat" in them.

It was necessary for him to have an arterial balloon procedure
(angioplasty). Though the procedure was successful, Bob didn't
bounce back as he usually did. Betty said he had the motivation
but not the energy or mental stamina to get going again. He became sluggish, had even more difficulty remembering simple
things. Since he was a diabetic, further testing seem feasible.

After weeks of exhaustive tests and diagnostic studies the con-
clusion was that Bob had Alzheimer's disease. Of course that
thought had entered his mind but only briefly considering his general good health and his active mind.

The day the Davises went to the doctor's office to hear the results of the tests was the beginning of the unbelievable, nightmarish road ahead of them. The doctor tried to prepare them for the news by telling them that he didn't have good news. They admitted they had already suspected that. Bob remarked that he had imagined all sorts of things from cancer to whatever. The doctor said, "I'd feel better if I could say you have cancer. . . . The tests have concluded that you have Alzheimer's disease."

The days that followed were filled with questions and struggles as they went through denial, anger, grief, and even "talking back" to God. Surely there was some mistake! But in time the recurring episodes of mental confusion proved the doctors were right. For the sake of the church and his own peace of mind, Bob knew that he had to give up his ministry. He really could not look after the flock as he wanted to and he wanted to bow out now—gracefully.

His congregation knew of his failing health but were nevertheless shocked at his announcement of retiring on August 2, 1987. It was a highly emotional moment as his members listened and wept as he said, "A Christian can do nothing greater than surrender completely to the Saviour. My life is not mine but Christ's.

"Today my ministry draws to a close, and I can say with the apostle Paul: 'I have finished the race, I have kept the faith.' Now I stand at the finish line in victory, because God himself set the distance I must run. . . .

"The greatest fear I have is what this disease does to your personality. It can make you angry, ugly, obscene, paranoid, cursing, and very difficult to handle before you become comatose. Pray that I be spared part of this personality change. Pray that I in no way inadvertently disgrace the Lord, this church, or the people whom I love.

"Pray for Betty, as I turn guardianship over to her. I will not suffer nearly as much as she will.

"And please have patience with me. At times my mind may not function. When it happens, remember that Bob Davis doesn't live in this body anymore. Please remember me the way I was.

"Finally, when I get to that stage where my mind is gone, pray the Lord will just take me home quickly. The glory of being with Jesus makes me gasp for joy."

There were times when the Davises asked, "Isn't God in charge? What did we do to deserve this? Doctors are only human—surely they made a mistake." Bob was a man of the Scriptures so he knew it was fruitless to ask "Why?" God's sovereignty over His creation does not yield to mere mortals' questions.

As confusion began to take over every day for Bob, he described it like this: "It's like sitting in front of a giant telephone switchboard, and no matter where you put the plug, you can't get an answer," he says. "I can look right at someone I know perfectly well or work with something familiar, but the name and the facts just aren't there. All the pictures stored away in the mind disappear. I can't even remember what my mother looked like."

A year later Bob could still converse sensibly so long as Betty was there to help him when his mind hit a snag. He now wears dark glasses, even inside, to block out some of the stimuli that tend to confuse him.

Betty says he continues to pray daily that the Lord will not allow his personality to deteriorate, causing him to become hostile and sullen. No sign of that has appeared.

As soon as Bob resigned, the Davises took care of all legal matters so Bob could participate in the decisions. Betty says they are prepared for the worst, while living in expectation of the best.

Even in this mental state, Bob Davis's life and work stand as a testimony in the community and surrounding areas. His last dramatic service had a tremendous effect on the community. One fellow pastor said that Bob had made a tremendous impact for Christ when he was healthy, but his witness went national when he got this awful disease.

The Davises were overwhelmed by the love and concern displayed in the community. Betty says with all the offers of help that came, they had to be careful that well-meaning friends didn't frustrate them. They had decided to leave all of it in the hands of the physicians whom they trust as God's instruments, confident that God will show His will.

When Bob was asked about faith healing, he spoke very slowly concentrating upon each word. "Well, we all want magic, I guess. But the Lord made it clear to me I'm no different from Paul the apostle. You remember he prayed three times for . . . whatever it was to be removed, but it wasn't. Yet he was able to say . . . what was it he said, Betty?"

"I have learned, in whatsoever state I am, therewith to be content," she said matter-of-factly .

Bob continued, " . . . now we know personally that God loves us in bad times as well as in good times—in sickness and in health. We're nothing more than his lambs, and he holds us to his breast."

Bob left the room for a moment and returned with a picture of Jesus holding a lamb. It seemed the lamb was thinking how good and safe it was in the arms of Jesus.

As tears slipped from behind the dark glasses, Bob says, "A beautiful lady in our congregation gave me that picture. She takes care of retarded children." As his words faltered Betty picked up for him, "She surely knew we were going through our darkest spiritual experience. Bob couldn't remember Bible verses, couldn't preach, and couldn't explain the Gospel anymore. He'd always had closeness with the Holy Spirit, but somehow that was gone too. In its place were horrible fears—even hallucinations. That picture arrived when all our 'Why, God?' questions were bombarding heaven."

The former pastor and gridiron star wiped his eyes. "The picture gives the only possible answer to all those questions," he said. "It seemed as though the lamb was showing me how it should be done." Bob smiled, relishing the memory. "I don't have to know any more about all this than the lamb knows. I am just as safe as he is, whatever my circumstances."

Betty agreed and nodded, "This hasn't turned out to be a story of faith healing. It's a story of faith acceptance. Our learning to accept God's will is just as great a miracle."[10]

17

The Nursing Home Quandary

If I may paraphrase Shakespeare, "To commit, or not to commit; that is the question!" This is the question too many of us have had to answer or are trying to settle now. I am positive it must be one of life's roughest decisions. It calls up emotions in us that are painful and even sickening. It goes against everything we have ever thought we would do. Remember feeling and believing that our parent or spouse would never be subjected to an institution for long-term care? To those of us who have been there, we understand your anxiety, your depression, your guilt, anger, fatigue, feelings of hopelessness and helplessness. I understand how you may wake up in the middle of the night in a cold sweat overwhelmed by frustration—trying to choose between the infirm family member and your children and spouse, or the infirm member and your own health and sanity. I know what it is to long for the comfortable time in your life when there was warmth and unafflicted love and the most pressing priority in life was how to get all the housework done or even all the monthly bills paid. But these feelings are heavy and won't go away.

Perhaps the first question to be settled in a family's mind is whether to send a family member to a nursing home or some other long-term facility. Is this a consideration because of your own health and the continuation of a normal home life for those left there? Has this come as a suggestion from your physician? If the parent or spouse is competent, how does he feel about institutional living? Can he adapt? How much input should he have? What if it doesn't work out? Can you bring him or her back home again? What will your neighbors and church friends think? Will they think you are just shirking your responsibility? If there is criticism, can you emotionally handle that?

How about the financial situation? Can Mother afford to live in an institution? Have you looked into what she is eligible for from Medicare or Medicaid? Are you aware that practically all of her means will be depleted before she is eligible for real financial aid at the nursing home from Medicaid? Is your family willing to "give up their inheritance" from Mother to have it spent on long-term nursing care? On the other hand, how much assistance is the primary caregiver receiving from other members of the family who are "against putting Mother away"? How often are they coming around to see Mother now? Be assured they will not visit her in the nursing home that often but they will probably be quick to remind you that they were opposed to her being there in the first place. Whatever your decision or your family's decision is, you won't please everyone —family or friends. Are there alternatives to consider instead of the usual nursing home?

I have been thrilled and surprised to find some of the alternatives to the conventional nursing homes. Nancy Fox in her book *you, your parent, and the nursing home* ("The Family's Guide of Long-term Care") suggests a number of alternatives to try before deciding on an institution.

These alternatives are called community services: home health-care services, day-care centers, night-sitters, grocery deliveries, volunteer visitors, dial-a-ride, meals-on-wheels, telephone reassurance, homemakers' services, physician visits, visiting nurses, mental-health counseling, home therapy, senior centers, family-respite service, share-a-home, foster home, supervised apartment, retirement home, assistance from friends and neighbors, and hospices.[1]

Of course, all of these services are not available in every community, but many are. Check with Information and Referral Service in the telephone book for what is available in your community, or call the Area Agency on Aging or the Council for the Aging.

Don't wait until you need to make a change to begin to look around for alternatives. Give yourself plenty of time to investigate thoroughly what is out there. In some instances, you will be completely turned off by what you find. You will know immediately this place is not for Mother or Dad and will look elsewhere. Perhaps in some places you will feel that the care would be adequate but the icy feeling that nobody really cares or is aware of needs around them pervades the place. Everything appears to be a job with personnel but with little feeling and warmth. Many older people are like children. Touching is more important than medication or food. To have someone acknowledge that one is a person with feelings and intelligence restores some of the dignity that may have been lost.

Most of the alternatives I have mentioned allow the elderly to maintain their independence and their dignity. When a person is mentally competent, many of the alternatives might be a possibility. Sharing a home seems to be a popular and satisfying arrangement for a number of seniors. They try to look after each other. What one cannot do or cares not to do, another will. Maybe one person loves to garden or work in the flowers while another prefers working inside and cooking. Cleaning services that come to the home on a weekly or biweekly basis can be the answer to house cleaning with expenses being shared equally. It is very important for each resident in a shared-living arrangement to have a room and, hopefully, a bath by himself. We all need space by ourselves to be able to think, pray, write, or do other private things that mean so much to us. Needless to say, it is important for all the residents of such a house to be congenial and willing to carry his or her share of the load financially and as much as possible physically. Living together in this manner also provides company and safety for the residents in more of a familylike setting.

Many families are finding that adult day-care centers are meeting a real need in their family's life. It is not uncommon for the college-age child to drop Grandmother off at the center as he or she goes to classes because Mother and Dad have long since gone to work. Perhaps another family member picks Grandmother up at the end of the day. Arrangements also might be made with a stay-at-home mother who has small children to take care of Grandmother during the day. All possibilities need to be explored before an institution is decided on. It goes without saying that the mental capabilities of the one needing care determines to a great degree the kind of care available.

Finding a live-in companion is ideal but is difficult and usually very expensive. I doubt, however, that it is more expensive than nursing-home care, and it certainly is more satisfactory to the one being cared for. What a comfort to be able to be surrounded by all the things one has collected, used, loved, and shared through the years with family and friends. I personally believe life is extended by avoiding the trauma associated with moving out of one's long-time home. Finding the correct, reliable person is the key to this arrangement.

Some share-a-homes might be on the order of a room-and-board type facility where there would be an administrator-type person who oversees all the housekeeping details but no nursing care is given. Each resident probably would have her own room or suite and would live quite independently, but the meals would be prepared and served in a common dining room and housekeeping service would be provided for the rooms or suites. This is much on the order of some lovely retirement facilities now in existence. This seems to be quite satisfactory for many people. Here again, cost is a factor which must be considered.

One dear lady who recently lost her husband wants to remain in her own rural home but is negligent about cooking and eating when she is alone. The family has arranged for a niece to stay with her during the day so that she will feel obligated to cook lunch for the niece and, therefore, eat. The widow prefers to stay alone at night. So far this is working well for this family. We have to be ingenious and look for creative ways to meet the needs of all family members. The caregiver family should not feel guilty over doing what seems best for their individual circumstances.

When parents have to move from the family home into other facilities, regardless of what they are, it is very traumatic. They see their cherished things being distributed to others who lack the emotional attachment they have. They fear that they will never have their "things" together again. They realize that they probably will never live in this house again and all they will really be able to take with them are the memories.

Early one Saturday morning as I was walking my three miles, I came upon a garage sale. I stopped out of curiosity to look over the pitiful offering of many years of frugal housekeeping. In the door of the house was a tiny old woman with the saddest look on her face. She watched as strangers pawed over her "things" and bargained with a younger couple for the well-worn appliances, dishes, and such that had been hers for many years. I have carried with me that mental picture of the little woman with a broken heart, who was apparently leaving under duress. A realtor's sign was in the front yard with a superimposed *SOLD* over it. I walked on with a sad heart asking myself the question, *Will I be that little old woman one day?* I pray not! The anguish of breaking up a home is not only real to the older folk but to the children and grandchildren. There is something so special about "going home" or going to Grandma's house on holidays. Preserving the memories for all the family members is no little thing. I was an only granddaughter on either side of the family for twenty-one years so I know about it firsthand. My only surviving grandmother and I had a very special relationship.

Nancy Fox, whose book I mentioned earlier, suggests that "the nursing home is a good idea for parents only if all the other options have been tried and exhausted and only if family circumstances are such that home care or alternatives constitute too great a physical and emotional burden on the family. In short, for your parent, the nursing home must be the last resort.

Let's define the types of available care at most present-day nursing home. There are facilities that do not offer all of these options but this is one of those things that must be looked into before admitting a loved one.

Custodial care: If a resident is continent, needs help only with meals, occasional dressing and bathing, and safety from the usual mishaps that occur when one lives alone, for example, then custodial care ("light care") from unskilled personnel is all that is required.

Intermediate care: This type of care must be provided by a state licensed facility that provides on a regular basis health care and services to those who need a degree of care and treatment. This facility provides more than room and board; they also provide special diets, simple medical procedures and injections, uncomplicated dressings, therapy, and exercise. Usually this care provides for at least one registered nurse to supervise such things as injections and medicines but probably will be staffed primarily by nursing assistants or licensed practical/vocational nurses.

Skilled care: This type of care is provided on an in-patient basis and requires more skilled nursing personnel. This may involve rehabilitation and restorative services, including inhalation therapy, drug therapy, occupational therapy and/or the administration of intravenous fluids. Most often these patients are bedfast or near so and need constant, close supervision.

Beginning October 1, 1990, the distinction between skilled level of care and intermediate level was erased. Residents are now cared for based on their individual needs, and the Medicaid/Medicare programs will reimburse nursing homes based on those care needs. This change should make it easier to find nursing home placement for "heavy care" patients. This action is another provision of the Nursing Home Reform Bill (OBRA '87).[2]

I want to borrow again from Nancy Fox's book *you, your parent, and the nursing home,* the material on how to select the right nursing home and the accompanying comparison checklist, pages 32 and following.

How to Select the Right Nursing Home

1 Obtain a catalog of nursing homes from your state department of health.

2. Shop well in advance for a home so that this is not a time-pressured, crisis-burdened choice.

3. Visit a home without prior appointment. Ideally, make several such visits to a home that appeals to you, making your visits at different times of the day, even at night.

4. The Freedom of Information Act has established the right of public access to nursing home inspection reports, on file in any district Social Security office. Take time to check these out. For Medicare facilities, provider survey reports and statements are filed. Medicaid approved homes are listed at the county department of social services.

5. In considering a particular home, ask the health department whether this home has ever received an "Intent to Deny License" because of uncorrected sanitary, fire, and/or patient care deficiencies.

6. State licensure does not necessarily indicate adequate inspection systems. When was the last inspection made? By whom? With prior appointment? What qualifications did the inspectors have? Answers to such questions may be found through consumer-advocate groups, your state ombudsman, or other concerned agencies.

When a family begins the search for a nursing home, it would be wise to check several and compare. If the answer to any of these questions is no, then you should have serious doubts about that home. (This compilation is in large part based on a government checklist.)

Initial Questions

—Does the home have a current state license on display?
—Does the administrator have a current state license?
—Does the home have a history of serious violations from state reports?

—Is the home certified to participate in financial assistance programs?
—Do current residents seem happy within the facility?
—Have they meaningful ways to occupy their time?

Location

—Is the home near a hospital?
—Is it convenient to family and friends?
—Is it convenient for the patient's physician?

Residents

—Is a Patients' Bill of Rights posted in plain sight for all residents?
—Do residents have the right to speak and associate freely?
—Are they free to complain without retaliation?
—May they receive visitors?
—Are patients encouraged to vote in public elections?
—Do patients know where to make official complaints?
—Have they the right to worship freely?
—Are arrangements made for various religions?
—Is there no discrimination on the basis of race, creed, color, or national origin?
—Are patients used as test subjects only with their informed consent?
—Are physical restraints used only when ordered by a doctor and is duration of use frequently reviewed by that doctor?
—Is the right to privacy respected? Curtain around bed? Is it used?
—Is there a private telephone for patient use?
—Is there a place for private family visits? A privacy room?
—Are residents given reasonable freedom to decide "lights out" time (i.e., *not* "put to bed" at a child's early hour for staff convenience, then given sleeping pills)?

Administration

Does the administrator know most patients by name?

—Is the administrator available to answer questions, hear complaints, or discuss problems?

—Does the administrator spend most of his or her day at the facility?

—Are names and addresses of the owner and administrator available?

—Is the administrator courteous and helpful?

Nursing Services

—Is the facility adequately staffed day and night and on weekends?

—Is the staff turnover rate low? How many on the staff have been employed for over two years?

—Have adequate provisions been made for patient care during staff absence?

—Is a written patient-care policy kept current and available for each patient? Is it implemented?

—Are adequate records kept? (Check at your Social Security office.)

—Are thorough answers given to your questions?

—Is there a restorative nursing care program aimed at promoting independence?

—Are RNs and/or LPNs on duty day and night? Seven days a week?

—Is there an isolation room for patients with contagious diseases?

—Do residents' visitors and volunteers speak favorably about the home?

—Are nursing aides paid more than the minimum wage required by the government?

—Is prompt care for the incontinent provided? At no extra cost? (Only the use of certain special equipment warrants any extra charges.)

General Physical Considerations

—Is the home clean and orderly?

—Is it free of unpleasant odor?

—Are rooms well ventilated and kept at a comfortable temperature?

—Is the general atmosphere warm, pleasant, cheerful?

Safety

—Are wheelchair ramps provided wherever necessary, indoors as well as outside?

—Is the home free of hazards: obstacles to patients, unsteady chairs, underfoot hazards?

—Are there grab bars in toilet and bathing facilities, handrails on both sides of hallways?

—Is an escape plan posted in a conspicuous place showing all exits and traffic patterns in case of fire? In case of other emergency?

—Are exit doors marked and easily opened from the inside?

—Are stairways enclosed and doors kept closed?

—Are fire extinguishers checked annually?

—Are hallways and ramps wide enough for two wheelchairs to pass easily?

—Are warning signs posted for unavoidable hazards, such as wet floors?

—Are rooms free of electrical cords?

—Are doorway thresholds flat?

—Are there call buttons within reach in rooms and baths?

—Is the home well lighted by day and night? Well enough for residents to read?

—Do beds have side rails?

—Is the furniture sturdy?

—Are auxiliary lighting and power available for emergencies?

—Do bathtubs and showers have nonslip surfaces?

—Is there an automatic sprinkler system? Has it recently been checked?
—Are certain areas posted with "No Smoking"signs? Are these observed?

Medical Services

—Are there adequate emergency procedures with doctor, ambulance, and necessary equipment available?
—Is there a medical director employed at the home?
—Are patients seen by physician at least every thirty days for the first three months and at regular intervals after that?
—Is there a public telephone within reach of wheelchair patients?
—Is the name and telephone number of the medical director furnished to patients and relatives?
—Are relatives notified prior to patient relocation? Is patient's consent obtained, wherever possible, before relocation? Relatives' consent?
—Does the home have an arrangement with outside specialized services, such as for dental, hearing, eye, and foot care?
—Is there a substitute always available for attending physician in emergency?
—Does the doctor actually visit with the resident, answer questions, and give emotional support during visits?
—Are pharmaceutical services supervised by a qualified pharmacist?

Food Service

—Is licensed dietitian on the premises often enough to supervise adequately the planning and preparation of meals? (Ask to see the kitchen area in order to observe order and cleanliness.)
—Are meals varied, nutritious, appetizing, and served at appropriate temperatures?
—Are menus posted, and do meals conform to those menus?
—Are special diets available?
—Are religious dietary laws accommodated?

—Are meals served at appropriate intervals?

—Is plenty of time allowed for each meal?

—Are adequate utensils provided?

—Is prompt assistance given with eating when needed—at no ex tra cost?

Is the dining room attractive and comfortable? Are there numer ous small tables, rather than unsociable long ones?

Rehabilitation Activities

—Are evening as well as daytime activities scheduled?

—Are activities carried out as posted? Are field trips available?

Are many residents given the opportunity to par ticipate?

—Is there a large room available for special activities? (Check how often many residents take part in activities.)

—Are there group as well as individual activities?

—Are residents encouraged to participate—but not pushed?

—Is there a qualified recreational staff?

Therapy

—Is there a full-time program of physical therapy available? What percentage of residents take part?

—Are occupational and speech therapy, as well as names of thera pists, available for all who need them?

—Are social services available to aid patients and their families?

—Are mental-health services available for all who need them?

—Is there a varied program of recreational, cultural, and intellec tual activities?

—Are activities offered for those who are relatively inactive or confined to their beds?

—Are barbers, beauticians, and masseurs/masseuses avail able?

Finances

—Is a written statement provided which details what is and what is not included in the daily rate?
—Is an itemized bill provided each month?
—Will the administrator give an estimated total monthly cost for an individual patient?
—Are there services which require extra charges?
—Are payment plans available and explained?
—Is a deposit required?
—Does the home have an adequate financial base?
—Is bonding provided for patient money?
—Are there adequate safeguards for patient's money and valuables? (Actually, it is best to take these home— watches, rings, etc.)
—Is there an adequate policy to compensate for personal possessions lost or stolen?
—Does the home concur that relatives need to bring an attorney when signing contracts?

Other Areas of the Home

—Does the home have an outdoor area where residents can get fresh air and sunshine? Is it often used?
—Is there a lounge where patients can read, chat, play games, watch TV, or just relax—away from their rooms?
—Are visiting hours convenient for patients and visitors?[3]

If a nursing home tested on the above questions scores high, in all probability you will have found a place you and your loved one can feel good about.

All nursing homes in our country either are operated for profit (proprietary) or are nonprofit (church, fraternal, or government sponsored). For a list of nursing homes in your area, write to your state department of health; to the American Health Care Association, 1200 Fifteenth Street, Washington, DC 20005, which represents the for-profit homes; or to the American Association of

Homes for the Aging, 1050 Seventeenth Street, Washington, DC 20036, which represents the nonprofit homes.

In addition to the questions listed above, I'd like to share, with her permission, some additional suggestions and observations made by our local nursing-home ombudsman, Kathy Gannoe. Nursing homes are in business to make money. True, they have certain state and federal guidelines by which they must operate but the bottom line is making a profit. If patients cannot pay their own way, their choices are limited about which nursing home they will use because many will not accept Medicaid patients. The reason is simple: a home receives about 20 percent less from Medicaid patients than they do from private-pay patients, and they reserve a sizable number of beds for those patients. While the law requires that there be no discrimination in the care administered, the home reserves the right to "determine" if they can provide the kind of care a patient may need. For instance, a home might tell the family they cannot give Aunt Suzie the care she needs. What they don't say is that since Aunt Suzie weighs 275 pounds, has a bedsore and is not mobile, they cannot take her because caring for her would require the use of a Hoyer turning device. OSHA now says the home must have three persons to operate the Hoyer and that would mean adding another employee, which would drastically impact the bottom line—profit. It sometimes seems that if a person has money, he or she can get into most any nursing home.

It is well to choose a nursing home near your usual route of travel so the family can drop in more often. A five-minute visit several times a week is better than a two-hour visit once a week. This gives the resident an opportunity of seeing the family frequently and though the visit isn't long, it says he is thought of and cared for. The family member has less guilt and is therefore more cheerful and isn't carrying around the resentment of having to visit. This also gives the nursing home the idea they never know when you might drop in. Try going at 5:00 p.m. on Saturday or 9:00 a.m. on a three-day weekend. You can judge pretty well the kind of care your family member is receiving.

Nursing-home residents are very heterogeneous—they have little in common except age and illness. You will find social classes among the mentally alert. Kathy Gannoe calls them the filet-mignon-with-duchesse-potatoes set; meat-loaf-and-scalloped-potatoes group; and white-beans-and-corn-bread crowd. The classes are very distinct and obvious and this can add to the discomfort and isolation of a "poor" new resident. Sometimes the residents place themselves in these groups but often the children do, as they mention in the proper circles that "Mother is now living in a particular home."

Another status symbol in a nursing home is whether or not a resident has cognitive ability, is alert, and can communicate. If she is ambulatory and has visitors, then she is more likely to have status with administration and residents. Patients with status are at least risk for being abused as well. Regardless of where we are and whatever our circumstances, we tend to seek out our own kind.

One deterrent to good nursing-home care is the poorly trained personnel who give personal care to the patients. Many have little or no training; some have no respect or compassion for elderly people; others look at it as just a job and feel whatever they give is all the home and patient deserve since they are paid such a miserly wage, often no more than minimum. With the proper training and attitude, the nurse's aide or nursing assistant can make all the difference in the outlook of the patient.

Many residents feel as if they have been abandoned by their families and that no one cares anymore. They feel they have been thrown into the hands of strangers who do not see them as people wanting to live out the remainder of their days in dignity and happiness but rather as the tail end of life who has come to this place to wait to die. And, with this attitude, often it isn't long until they do die. In fact, the average life span of a nursing home resident is only 2.4 years.

Can we visualize how we would react if we were physically and mentally unable to care for ourselves; sick, weak, and yes, scared, feeling abandoned by the people we have loved and cared for all these years? Suddenly, we are stripped of our home and surroundings and those things that are familiar. We have had to leave our watch, jewelry, and perhaps even our wedding band at home because the likelihood of their being stolen is too great.

We've even lost our names! We are referred to as "dearie" "sweetheart" or as twenty-five or fifty-one, referring to our room number. Most elderly persons don't even want to be called by their first names by strangers who have not asked permission. It is very depersonalizing to lose one's name. We need to remember that, most of the time, these patients are just like the rest of us but trapped in a body that is wearing out. They don't want to be treated like a child by personnel who use baby talk or patronizing gestures.

Mentally healthy residents need to make as many decisions and be involved in all decision-making processes as far as is possible for a continued sense of independence. Unfortunately, in too many long-term care facilities, someone else makes all the decisions. The resident is told when to get up, when to get a bath, when to eat, when to put on a sweater, when to go to chapel, when to take medicine, when to go to the bathroom, and when to go to bed. Often, a home will be so short staffed that everything is regimented to allow the staff to get it all done. Having less staff also means more profit for the owner in the "for-profit" homes.

Numerous other cuts are made in many homes to save money and short-circuit the care given to patients, thus increasing the profit for the "often absent owner" who is involved in other businesses.

Abuses of residents in nursing homes began coming to the attention of the media and ultimately to Congress several years ago. Even though federal legislation was passed some time ago to stop nursing home abuse, it still exists and may be getting worse. Most of the states are dragging their feet at implementing this legislation. One problem with closing down a nursing home is what to do with the residents. Many would have nowhere else to go. They can't just be thrust out into the street.

In 1980, the *Louisville* (Ky.) *Courier-Journal* ran a series of articles about the physical and mental abuse in nursing homes. Reports of patients being pinched, hit, denied supper or other meals, being thirsty in the middle of the night and being denied water or having their hair pulled, appeared to be common "discipline" for those who wet the floor, refused to take their medicine, or otherwise refused to cooperate with the establishment.[4] Accounts are reported of nursing-home staff bringing a tray to a blind person who is napping and never telling him the food is there or putting it out of his reach and taking it away before he has a chance to eat. Or a patient lies wet and soiled for hours in a cold room until finally someone comes to change the bed but ridicules the patient for what he has done, holding the soiled linens under his nose to shame him or her. One patient was tied on the toilet seat and fed her supper because she often wet the dining-room floor. This way, if she needed to urinate, she would be in the appropriate place, so said the administrator.

Art Linkletter in his book *Old Age Is Not for Sissies* tells where a patient's head was held under water until he stopped struggling against the aide who was trying to bathe him; of patients being slapped for not answering a question; being drugged to the point that they cannot object to anything that goes on; being deliberately dropped, beaten, or other-wise roughed up—even raped.[5] Are you also appalled at the mistreatment of these old, sick, frail, maybe blind, deaf, or mentally disoriented elderly people?

Not answering the call bell is a common practice in some substandard homes. It is true that many patients constantly call for nurses, but how can one distinguish a genuine call from someone just wanting attention? Family members might find their loved ones soiled and wet, obviously for hours. This is blatant neglect. The series in the *Louisville Courier-Journal* gave blow-by-blow descriptions of bedsores patients were allowed to develop. Bedsores develop when prolonged pressure is put on the skin and causes it to break down. The best way to avoid them, doctors say, is to turn patients frequently. Naturally this requires more staff and closer supervision of patients, thus costing the home more money. Bed-sores are extremely difficult to heal and, if left untreated, can cause death through infection.

Once more, the attitude of the staff makes all the difference. Too frequently, staff views these people as those waiting their turn to die and give another unfortunate soul their bed. In some documented cases, staff has been slow or failed altogether to call a doctor when a patient is choking or has had a near-fatal accident. It is true that some patients complain often and demand that the doctor be called, but there are times when the patient really does need a doctor.

Some nursing homes are closed because they were not giving the residents enough to eat. The portions were too small and nutritionally deficient. The reporter described the dinner scene with residents "literally licking crumbs from each other's trays and from off the bare table," because they were so very hungry. Have you ever noticed how the food is plopped down in one of those little recesses in the food trays in most nursing homes? Often those who wait tables further insult the dignity of the residents by carelessly bringing in the trays so that foods run from one section to another. This is quite a change if the resident has been accustomed to having dinner with a family whose dinner table was covered with a cloth and fabric napkins were used; where food was passed and served with pride and interest. Some nursing homes are getting their patients up at the crack of dawn, 5:30, and serve breakfast at 6:30 and then dinner at 4:30 (so the dining room staff can get home in time to take care of their own families). The reasoning behind this is, "what difference does it make, they (the patients) aren't going anywhere, so one time is as good as another." Most nursing home residents have arthritis and getting out of bed early in the morning can be a painful task. To be yanked out and immediately pushed to begin a routine such as breakfast, baths, or exercise is just too much for an elderly person. Some homes are so regimented that the routine is more important than the patient.

It is natural to ask why these conditions and many others that

have not been enumerated, exist. The answer is always one word
—*money*. There aren't enough federal dollars for Medicare and
Medicaid patients and a moderately well-off family is soon broke
because many homes cost more than $2,000 per month. Medicare,
the federal program designed to provide for the health-care needs
of Americans over age sixty-five, provides little coverage of the
cost of long-term care, actually only 100 days per year of hospital
stay. All Americans over the age sixty-five are eligible for Medicare, regardless of income, but it pays limited amounts even for
community-based, long-term care services.[6]

Medicaid is a federal-state matching program providing medical assistance for certain low-income persons. Each state administers its own program and determines the eligibility and scope of
benefits, subject to federal guidelines. The Federal Government's
share of medical expenses is tied to a formula based on the per-
capita income of the state.[7]

Each state designs and administers its own Medicaid program
within broad federal guidelines. As a result, there are significant
variations among states with regard to eligibility requirements,
benefits provided, and provider reimbursement policies.[8]

Unfortunately, one must either be very poor to start with or
have already spent down his or her income or savings to the eligibility level of a specific state in order to be eligible for Medicaid.

Families should thoroughly check with their local Department
of Health and Human Services about services and assistance available through Medicaid. Often, nursing-home residents must use
all their resources and those of a spouse before they are eligible. In
other words, a person can't be eligible for Medicaid until he is
poor—either has always been poor, or be the "new poor" because
all resources have been spent earlier on services.

Can you imagine the additional worry an ill person will have
knowing his life savings are slipping away like sand through his
fingers? What a blow to the dignity and feeling of self-sufficiency

of an elderly person! It is only natural for the patient to be concerned about his spouse and what will happen to him or her financially in the future. Doubtless, this hastens the demise of a patient.

Our country is faced with a world-sized dilemma about health costs and care for all Americans, but especially the elderly.

More than one-half of the elderly couples are impoverished after one spouse has spent only six months in a nursing home. Most often, it is the wife who remains in the community, and she often is left with little or no money with which to meet her own health and other needs. A couple is allowed to keep their home because the government reasons that if the patient should get well enough to go home, he would need a home and not become homeless. Additionally, a small amount is allowed the spouse in a savings account and a small amount per month for the spouse at home, if she has no income in her own name. It is hardly enough to pay for shelter and utilities. The spouse in the nursing home is allowed a minimum amount for personal needs—clothes, phone calls, personal care such as the barber shop, and recreational expenses.[9]

Elderly persons are slightly more likely than other adults to be poor. Older women in every age group are substantially more likely to be poor than men of the same age. In 1984 women accounted for more than half of the elderly population; they accounted for nearly three-fourths of the elderly poor.[10]

Generally, when determining Medicaid eligibility, income (such as Social Security checks, pensions, and interest from investments) is attributed to the person whose name is on the instrument conveying the funds. In the case of Social Security, the amount attributed to each spouse is the individual's share of the couple's benefit. Therefore, if the couple's pension check is made out to the husband, all of that income is considered his for the purpose of determining Medicaid eligibility. Because the current generation of women whose husbands are at risk of needing nursing home care typically did not work outside the home, they likely have very little income other than their husband's.

The attribution of resources such as certificates of deposit and savings accounts is done similarly. If the resources are held solely by the institutionalized spouse, they are attributed to him or her for purposes of determining Medicaid eligibility. If they are in both spouses' names, they are still attributed to the institutionalized spouse. Medicaid eligibility can be denied to individuals who transferred resources for less than fair market value within two years of applying for Medicaid. Once an institutionalized spouse has been determined to be Medicaid eligible, some of his monthly income is reserved for the use of his spouse. When combined with the spouse's income (if one exists), it allows a maintenance needs level. Maintenance needs levels vary from state to state.[11]

(Developments in Aging: 1987, Volume 3, "The Long Term Care Challenge." A report of the Special Committee on Aging, US Senate, Pursuant to S. RES. 80, Sec. 19, January 28, 1987. Resolution Authorizing a Study of the Problems of the Aged and Aging. US Government Printing Office, Washington: 1988.)

In nursing home or long-term care facilities that accept federal monies as well as private paying patients, the care must by law be the same care. Therefore, patients and staff are not supposed to know who is private pay and who is Medicaid assisted. Of course, the administration has access to those records. But, if an institution does not accept federal monies and a patient's funds run out, then he or she is out on her ear, so as to speak.

Fortunately, the public now has an ally to assist them in correcting or improving nursing-home conditions. That is the nursing home ombudsmen in your area and each state has at least one. Most states have several who are assigned a given number of nursing homes in an area. I am again indebted to Art Linkletter in his previously mentioned book for defining the word *ombudsman*, which he says dates back to the fifteenth century and is a Scandinavian word that literally means "for the people." Perhaps the following paragraph from his book will better define the word as he allows a woman who has been an ombudsman for a number of years to describe herself.

"We're the people who everyone hiding something hates: the

agencies who may not be doing their jobs, the institutions or facilities that have something to hide, and family members abusing someone inside or outside a nursing home." She went on to say that an ombudsman gets treated with a lot of respect when people discover that the law in some states includes the possibility of felony convictions that carry a $10,000 fine and/or a two-year prison term for those convicted of abuse; the same fine can be also meted out to those who observe abuse and do not report it. Their authority extends also to hospitals, group homes, home-care agencies, families, and state agencies. He or she can cause a facility to be shut down.[12]

From what I have shared with you, it would appear that I think all nursing homes are bad and a poor choice for your loved one. This is not my intent; rather it is to encourage families and caregivers to explore every avenue to find the very best facility for their family member. Read everything you can find, talk to people, go look for yourself—don't take someone else's word for it. Do it early before a pressing need arises, and the pressure of the moment forces settling for less than the best for your situation.

Through the years most of us have become attached to our physician to some degree. From time to time we have been reassured by him, we have had bad news broken gently (by most doctors, anyway), we have come to look at him as a barometer of our health—one who will tell it like it is, one we can trust, and one who has taken a personal interest in us and our physical condition. Fortunate indeed is the patient who can retain his own physician when he enters a long-term care facility. However, not all nursing homes allow this and often a patient must take a doctor who is "assigned" or retained by that home to look after all the patients. This is one of those questions that should be asked before a patient is admitted.

If the nursing home is certified to take Medicare/ Medicaid patients, then the physician is required to visit every thirty days for skilled-care patients and every sixty days for intermediate-care patients. To meet this federal requirement, doctors have been known to just show up and look over a large group of people (Nancy Fox calls this "gang visiting") without really examining any of them and prescribe just about anything for them from tranquilizers to laxatives. Some just stick their heads in the door of the room and ask, "How're you feeling today, Mary? You're looking better. You behave yourself, now and I'll see you soon." One nurse calls this kind "doorsill doctors." Another doctor may respond to a complaint from a patient with such remarks as, "Well, you know that comes with old age, Sam. What can you expect at this time in your life?" Nothing is so depressing at any age as to be reminded how old we are and to attribute that physical condition at that time in our life to our age.

Maybe we would like to ask the question, "Why do these doctors agree to the care of these patients if they do not have compassion for geriatrics?" The answer is simple: money—mine and yours via Uncle Sam. Many doctors have been accused of ripping off the government of Medicare/Medicaid payments. And who has to verify and check the amount of time spent with a patient in a nursing home? Nobody! If a doctor recommends a certain nursing home, saying he can arrange right away for you to get your parent in—beware! He or she may own the home or have a substantial financial interest in it.

Fortunately, most physicians are not like I have described; but plenty do exist.

We were most fortunate in the care of my mother-in-law because we were able to retain the physician who had cared for her and diagnosed her condition. Max Crocker was not only a wonderful doctor but a great Christian with integrity who was genuinely interested in Mrs. Sisk. Our visits to the nursing home never coincided with his but nearly every time after he had made a home visit, he would take the time to call us personally and give us his evaluation of her condition and his recommendations. George Bernard Shaw is reported to have said, "Let no one suppose that the words 'doctor' and 'patient' can disguise the fact that they are employee and employer."

Sometimes we use the expression that so and so has become a grouchy, crabby old man or woman. In the majority of cases, elderly people have the same kind of personality they had when they were younger. The difference may be that when they were younger they realized how distasteful some of their attitudes were to others, so they tried to cover up or control such things as their tempers and a caustic tongue. Many times people revert to doing the things they once did when younger. Often the fear of life being nearly over, loneliness and isolation from having been widowed, dread of a devastating illness, or any number of disturbing things can make the worst in people come to the surface.

Kathy Gannoe, nursing home ombudsman for our area of Kentucky, has shared much of her materials for my research, including a video entitled, "What Do You See, Nurse?"[13] The script was very close to the following poem that was found among the possessions of an old Irish lady who had died in a geriatric hospital. The poem so impressed Betha Rainey, a young nurse on the hospital staff, that she sent the copy to the editor of *Beacon House News*, the magazine of the Northern Ireland Association for Mental Health. The poem gives a deep insight into how patients react to the care and attention of all staff with whom they come in contact at the hospital, and in particular, it illustrates the effect of their attitudes. I use this by courtesy of Kentucky Association of Mental Health.

Crabbit Old Woman

What do you see, Nurses, what do you see?
What are you thinking when you look at me?
A crabbit old woman, not very wise
Uncertain of habit, with far-away eyes?
Who dribbles her food and makes not reply
When you say in a loud voice, "I do wish you'd try!"
Who seems not to notice the things that you do.
And forever is losing a stocking or shoe
Who, unresisting or not, lets you do as you will

With bathing and feeding, the long day to fill.
Is that what you're thinking, is that what you see?
Then open your eyes, you're not looking at me.
I'll tell you who I am as I sit here so still
As I move at your bidding, as I eat at your will
I'm a small child of ten with a father and mother
Brothers and sisters who love one another
A young girl of sixteen with wings on her feet
Dreaming that soon now a lover she'll meet;
A bride soon at twenty—my heart gives a leap
Remembering the vows that I promised to keep;
At twenty-five now I have young of my own
Who needs me to build a secure happy home.
A woman of thirty my young now grow fast
Bound to each other with ties that should last.
At forty my young now will soon be gone
But my man stays beside me to see I don't mourn.
At fifty once more babies play round my knee.
Dark days are upon me, my husband is dead
I look at the future, I shudder with dread,
For my young are all busy rearing young of their own
And I think of the years and the love I have known.
I'm an old woman now and nature is cruel.
'Tis her jest to make old age look like a fool.
The body it crumbles, grace and vigor depart
And there's a stone where I once had a heart.
But inside this old carcass a young girl still dwells
And now and again my battered heart swells;
I remember the joys, I remember the pain
And I'm loving and living life over again.
I think of the years all too few—gone so fast
And accept the stark fact that nothing can last.
So open your eyes, Nurses, open and see
Not a crabbit old woman; look closer—see me.[14]

18

"I've Been There, Too"

Caregiving and the Sandwich Generation

Many of us leave this world the same way we came—with someone caring for us because we cannot care for ourselves. A tiny, newborn baby delights everyone and getting help to care for him is no problem. With joy parents watch their healthy children learn to do expected things at given ages. They keep a baby book, recording all these achievements, including date, place, situation, who saw it, and whether it was a feat that might say to the parents that they just might have a child prodigy. Pictures are made to send to grandparents and, in general, it is a happy moment of achievement.

Somewhere in time, at an age first undetermined, the scene changes. For some, it may be in the late forties but, generally speaking, for most it is late sixties. An older individual begins to show signs of really slowing down. Perhaps some years earlier he began to do those things he had never done before, like ride instead of walk when he played golf, walk instead of jog, or become a spectator of sports instead of an active participant. We consider this pretty normal, but there is no family member on the sidelines cheering him on as he relinquishes various activities. Little by little as the years pass, families realize this family member is getting older. There is no rejoicing but rather a sad, pitying feeling that he is in the sunset years of life.

We have not yet come to the place where we can view the end of life with the same joy and anticipation as the beginning. I wish I could, because I do have a Christian hope in Christ and I know that those who have that hope have eternal life with Christ. Knowing that our loved ones are with Him is a great comfort as we reluctantly give them up.

In the meantime, those in our families who have not reached that passage of life must be cared for, loved, and sometimes even protected—from themselves or from others. I have experienced those scenes I have just described to you. I wish the demise of a Christian were as joyous as the birth of a new baby.

Caregiving of our children is so wonderful and natural. We can hardly wait to advance from one stage to another. The vague thought of caring for elderly parents, an aunt or especially a spouse, is so far-fetched, we can't entertain such thoughts. For most of us, that time does come before we are ready for it or before we can believe it is happening.

Despite the rumor that Americans have, in most instances, abandoned their old folks, generally, this is not true! The family is still the primary caregiver of older Americans. Most older people live close to at least some of their children and have contact with them on a fairly regular basis. The National Institute on Aging reports that eight out of ten men and six out of ten women live in family settings.

Better Homes and Gardens magazine, November 1988, shared the results of a survey they did on some of the aspects of aging. One question was "What are your fears about growing old?" The results were: 68 percent said poor health/being unable to care for self, 41 percent said becoming a burden to spouse or children, 39 percent reported not enough money, and 22 percent said Alzheimer's disease; loneliness, senility, boredom, and being unable to keep their present home were others listed. Interestingly enough, 15 percent said they had no fears about growing old.

Another question was "What do you look forward to about growing older?" The answers were: 52 percent listed freedom to travel; 50 percent said spending more time with spouse; 46 percent named less stressful life-style; others listed more recreational time; perspective, wisdom, and understanding; financial security; time with grandchildren; and retirement. The answers also show that 14 percent did not look forward to growing old at all.

Another question was "If your elderly parent(s) became incapable of living alone, which alternative would you choose as the best solution for all concerned?" Parents moving into their child's home was named by 41 percent; 30 percent said a live-in helper in parent's home; a retirement home said 23 percent; a nursing home said 10 percent, and only 4 percent suggested a child move to the parent's home.

Additionally, from this report I share:

> With home, family, and neighbors being so cherished these days, 49% of our respondents plan to stay in their own home upon retirement. Says one: "We've worked all our lives for this place and we want to take the time to enjoy it." An additional 25% will continue living at home but spend part of the year elsewhere, 11% will move to a home or apartment in another community, 9% will move into a smaller home or apartment in the same community; a scant 3% say they plan to move to a retirement community.[1]

It seems that the preferences for types of care are changing as our communities are becoming more acutely aware of the plight of the elderly and the options open for their care. For instance, two decades ago, the nursing home was first choice but now by only 10 percent. In the early 1980s, cost was a primary concern but now people are more concerned about loneliness, despair, isolation, trauma for the elderly, and, in some instances, the possibility of some kinds of abuse in nursing homes.

Most of the elderly voice some fears and concerns. One fear is criminal acts against older people. In some communities, senior citizens are fearful of taking a walk, sitting on their porches after dark, or scolding children and youth who abuse their property for fear of reprisals. Cowardly criminals seem to seek out older, defenseless people and prey on them.

Falling is another fear the elderly have. Some can become almost paranoid about moving around freely even though they have never had a fall. Their lack of confidence makes them more likely to fall. This, of course, needs to be a concern but not a paralyzing one.

Many middle-aged and older people have an alarming fear of being institutionalized, as in a nursing home. Some say they feel they have little choice because they don't want to move in with any of their children. They admit they are afraid of various things and know they are getting forgetful, but the greatest fear is the nursing home.

One alternative to nursing homes is caring for the family member in the home of a relative—spouse, child, grandchild, niece, or nephew. Long before this need arises, the smart family will have had a meeting of family members who will or might be involved in the care of the individual. Another fear of the elderly is the loss of decision making regarding their welfare. It is important to involve the patient in this decision-making process if he is still mentally competent. When family members exclude the older person from what is being considered, it contributes to feelings of isolation and helplessness. An aged parent has both legal and moral rights to participate in decisions concerning his life.

Listen to what the older person has to say and try to understand his emotional needs. When an older person faces change, he experiences feelings of fear, anger, grief, and frustration. He fears the loss of home, independence, and place in the community. Let him express this to a sympathetic ear.

When the time comes to talk to your parent about making a change in life-style, the way you approach her will make a lot of difference. It is better to express your concern about her living alone, driving, or some other thing you feel she should give up than to use a command about what the parent must do. For example, "Mother, I'm concerned about your driving now," rather than, "Mother, you can't drive anymore—I want your car keys now!"

The decision about whom the parent will live with comes about in various ways. Statistics show that 85 to 95 percent of all caregiving is done by family members, mostly by a middle-aged daughter, whose average age is fifty-seven. More than a third of caregivers are over age sixty-five—one fourth were ages sixty-five to seventy-four, and 10 percent were seventy five or older. This means that informal services are largely provided by the "young old" to the "old old." She may be the only one nearby, she may be unmarried or not employed, she may volunteer, or she may more or less have it pushed on her by the other family members who begin making excuses why they can't—profession, small children, house too small, moving Mother from her familiar hometown, or "You were always Mother's favorite, I know she would want to live with you."[2]

According to the Older Women's League of America, more than 27 million days of unpaid care are provided for elderly folk each week. These days are provided by approximately 7 million Americans, mostly women, who toil without respite doing back-breaking labor in virtual isolation. Caregiving can be a financial, physical, and emotional burden for many mid-life and older women who are unable to find or afford help in caring for family members.

Frequently, caregiving starts out in assisting perhaps both parents in their own home with such things as driving them to the doctor, shopping, occasional cleaning and laundry, but not every day. As the health of one parent deteriorates and perhaps eventually dies or goes into long-term care, then the remaining one is unable to stay in the home. It is at this time that the family has to make crucial decisions about the care of the other parent (or other family member).

Ironically, it is not unheard of that the caregiver is never reimbursed for expenses she personally bore after long years of unpaid caring for an elderly parent and may be remembered to a lesser degree in the will or not at all, because she wouldn't allow Mother to drive the car, cook on the gas range, take night walks, or any other thing Mother wanted to do and couldn't.

Over the years, if there have been previous conflicts in the family between the parent (or spouse) and the caregiver, the stress and strain of this new arrangement will not help it and may even bring out old grudges and unforgiven incidents. If such a situation should exist, only the grace of God will see a family through this. It is difficult enough when there is genuine love, respect, and concentrated effort on everyone's part.

Why do we call these caregivers "the sandwich generation"? Because the elderly are living longer and many women are choosing to start their families later, they often have young children in the home. They may be professional or career women; and they are trying to care for an elderly or ailing parent. They are literally squeezed between these responsibilities like filling in a sandwich. They often feel as if they are in a vice with the very life being squeezed from them. Caught! The designated caregiver often feels fear, crushed dreams, doomed plans and expectations for later years, even helplessness, frustration, disbelief, anger, fatigue, guilt, and grief. Freedom to travel, do volunteer work, spend time with grandchildren, to paint or garden, or whatever dreams and plans had been made by a couple, seem so far away and unattainable at this time. Dwelling on these sacrifices can soon lead to caregiver depression and stress symptoms.

A typical day for such a caregiver might be to get up very early (maybe after having been up two or three times in the night to help Dad find the bathroom), get her own shower, and put on the day's makeup; get children up for school, get Dad up and help him dress; make breakfast for entire family; see that children have their books, lunch money, raincoats, and so forth, and are out the door in time to catch the bus (so she doesn't have to drive them to school); wash dishes, put in one load of laundry, help husband make beds; make sure Dad is dressed properly for the day; and then leave for work and day-care center to drop Dad off. Have a busy but pretty good day at the office but so nervous and tired, spill coffee on the front of a new dress early in day; have a silly confrontation with co-worker; pick up Dad from center; stop at grocery and dry cleaners; make dinner and clean up. Help Dad get bath and to bed but with resistance from him; help with homework; run sweeper in traffic lanes after kids were in bed. Fall into bed thoroughly exhausted; on the verge of tears; surely not interested in making love; feet that things have got to change but how, knowing the family can't make it on one salary if caregiver gives up job. This caregiver is sandwiched between several "slices of bread" and sees little hope of things changing soon. This is not an exaggerated example of a typical caregiver. It is true that not all female caregivers are employed, but you could describe your own scenario.

The primary caregiver, whether husband or wife, must have full support of a spouse before agreeing to care for an elderly family member. They need to sit down together privately and discuss how their home life will change, what plans will have to be "put on the back burner" and whether or not they can and are willing to make those changes. How much cooperation can the primary caregiver expect from a spouse? Is the relationship between an in-law and a daughter-in-law such that a long-term arrangement will work without the health of either deteriorating? Does the parent have sufficient funds to pay for some community services or domestic help and give the caregiver a respite from time to time? Would the parent be willing to spend his money that way? Could he see the need?

All these questions assume the patient is mentally competent. I personally feel that the funds of the ailing relative should be used to employ the help needed to care for him and to assist with the day-to-day chores and responsibilities of the household where he lives. Foods for a special diet and other incidentals that are required to give adequate care to the patient should be paid from their income or savings account. Caregivers should feel free to discuss the financial responsibilities with the competent patient and perhaps agree on how best to manage the funds. If funds are taken without prior agreement with the relative, it could lead to feelings of mistrust and apprehension. Keep everything open and above board as much as possible—all situations considered.

The most precious commodity we have is time. The realization that each ticking minute is taking us closer to our own demise and who knows what lies between now and then. To become a caregiver is giving one of life's most precious gifts—time. Another gift we give is energy. I doubt that any caregiver has had full comprehension of what was involved in time and energy when first she agreed to be a primary caregiver. On the average, caregivers help with four personal-care tasks: bathing, dressing, feeding, and taking one to the toilet. This often amounts to forty hours a week, sometimes more.

Each individual needs time for himself—to be by himself, to read, meditate, have some quality privacy, or do anything else that appeals to him. It needs to be unaccounted-for time, except with one's own conscience. We need the quietness and contemplation that is so necessary for our mental stability and strength. Time and energy may be the biggest sacrifices a caregiver is made to give.

Becoming a caregiver may be a threat to your mental stability. Can you stand hearing the same questions over and over all day long? Some experts in the field of geriatrics say the patient may be seeking contact and conversation but he may have lost the skills necessary for conversation or he may have a recent memory loss which prevents him from remembering or retrieving the information he has. Could you stand being followed around all day? He may feel insecure, or afraid of being lost or abandoned. It might help to place a special chair in the kitchen or den where he can see you and realize that you aren't going to leave him.

What will you do at the mall when he starts moaning and wringing his hands? Will you be embarrassed and leave as you did at church when he started rocking and wringing his hands or when you were at the grocery and he would not walk but would only clutch the cart and cry? Do you dare invite friends over not knowing what your parent will do or say? Can you then take the social isolation that you will feel you have to impose on yourself? I could list one scenario after another but could never cover all the possibilities. Much to the chagrin of most caregivers, patients are constantly coming up with actions, emotions, or questions that our minds just have not framed and often we are caught off guard and don't know how to cope or what to do.

All the above and much more causes untold stress on families. Many nursing-home admissions are the result of the primary caregiver being completely exhausted, ill, or stressed out from caring for the relative, so that the relative has to be admitted in order to save the caregiver.

To admit that you can't take it any longer brings untold guilt and worry. We are plagued with such thoughts as *She cared for me when I was a baby and unable to care for myself. She took care of me and my family when I was ill. She has given unselfishly to all of us through the years—doing without things herself, things that might seem like necessities to us today, in order for us to have some things we desired. Now when she is unable to care for herself any longer, we are about to make other arrangements.* During these stressful times we can't think straight. When our bodies are fatigued, so are our minds. Sometimes it becomes a juggling act for the caregiver as she tries to take care of too many people's needs.

Of necessity, there is housework, laundry, shopping, cooking, and nurturing other family members. Primary caregivers need to lower their own expectations and standards of housekeeping and meals. Decide privately, "How much am I willing to do? How much can I do?" Contract with your husband and children about their doing certain things to help and about their understanding of changes in the housekeeping routine. Maybe children have never changed their beds or cleaned their bathrooms. Ask them to take on that chore for you. Even small chores like pushing the garbage to the curb can seem like a tremendous help. Tell your husband that you would like him to be responsible for three meals a week and on those nights you will go to the nursing home to feed Aunt Tillie. Try to arrange with your children to stay home one night a week to sit with their grandfather so you can get out, if it is only to take a long walk. Secure contracts from siblings for certain things that will relieve a little pressure. When friends ask if there is anything they can do, tell them what would be helpful, being careful of course, not to take advantage of their offer (or they won't offer again). I am finding it much easier to tell you what to do than I found doing it, but I confess that my pride, my feeling of self-sufficiency probably kept me from enlisting more help. I didn't want to appear unable to handle any situation no matter how bad it was. We Christian women tend to layer too many things on ourselves in the way of expectations, feeling "with God's help, we can handle it!" And we do!

It is not uncommon to feel that we are neglecting our own children and spouse. Growing up through the teen years is so risky and trying, a family often feels they are walking on eggshells trying to get an adolescent through them. Children can so easily get hooked on drugs, alcohol, or other abusive things that families feel a particular obligation to give special attention to these young people. An already shaky marriage cannot take the stress and strain a caregiving situation imposes, and often ends in divorce. A caregiver feels pulled from one extreme to another trying to keep a family intact and give a parent or relative the care they need as well.

Parent Care, The University of Kansas Gerontology Center's January/February 1990 issue, suggests that patients have games they play with their caregivers.[3] It is not unusual for a frail elderly mother to try to control her middle-aged daughter by pretending to be more helpless than she really is. These are manipulative games they use to trick their caregivers into behaving the way they want. For instance, they use their age as an excuse to do or not to do something. They may also try feigning—going along with the caregiver's requests but appear to be having extreme difficulty carrying out their wishes. However, the older person has no problem doing things he chooses to do. He may want one thing but pretend it is something else. A parent who wants company may fake hunger or pain to get attention. The older person may reluctantly behave as the caregiver desires, but only when the caregiver is watching. Smoking or eating the wrong foods is a good example. He or she may have been told not go outside without the walker but they do when the caregiver's back is turned. Some parents may manipulate their adult children with physical symptoms. A mother may suddenly suffer from dizzy spells or heart palpitations whenever her daughter and son-in-law are planning a vacation, so they end up canceling their trip.

Caregivers need to be sure they are not sucked into this manipulation. Look for the source. Check all the physical symptoms; learn what is faked and what is genuine as much as possible. Gently but firmly remind the parent that you and your family have needs, too. Use humor when possible. Remind the parent that you do care but that you must take care of yourself so that you will be better able to care for her. Make adequate arrangements for her in your absence, then go ahead with your plans. If something should go wrong, refuse to take the blame or carry that load of guilt. Remember that you were honest with the parent and that you did what you thought best at the time. Older people, like children, can quickly pick up on our weaknesses and will often use them against us to have their own way.

Caregivers need to continue involvement in activities outside the home as much as possible, so as not to feel or become isolated from the world outside and even one's own family, who have outside interests. Family members should rotate caregiving responsibilities to help the primary caregiver and also to avoid dependency of the patient on the primary caregiver. If a household is small, the family might want to recruit live-in relatives or live-in hired help to give the primary caregiver some relief.

When you, the caregiver, feel angry or stressed, take a walk, if possible; talk it out with a friend or a counselor. When those guilt feelings hit, ask yourself, *Why am I feeling guilty? Should I? Have I done something that justifies this terrible feeling?* Don't wait until you reach the breaking point before you realize that something has to change. Listed below are some warning signs to take note of if you are a primary caregiver.

> Your relative's condition is worsening despite your best efforts.
> No matter what you do, it isn't enough.
> You feel you're the only person in the world enduring this.
> You no longer have any time or place to be alone for even a brief respite.
> Things you used to do occasionally to help out are now part of your daily routine.
> Family relationships are breaking down because of the caregiving pressures.
> Your caregiving duties are interfering with your work and social life to an unacceptable degree.
> You're going on in a no-win situation just to avoid admitting failure.
> You realize you're all alone and doing it all because you've shut out everyone who's offered help.
> You refuse to think of yourself because "that would be selfish" (even though you're unselfish 99 percent of the time).
> Your coping methods have become destructive: You're overeating/undereating, abusing drugs/alcohol, or taking it out on your relative or your family.
> There are no more happy times. Loving and caring have given way to exhaustion and resentment, and you no longer feel good about yourself or take pride in what you're doing. [4]

As a family (with or without the patient, depending on the mental condition), those concerned need to sit down and honestly and unemotionally as possible look at all the factors involved. The caregiver should openly and graphically explain to siblings or others involved just what the situation is and how you feel it is getting out of hand. Ask for suggestions and ideas as to what is the best course to take at this time. What other alternatives are open to the family? Explore each one thoroughly, considering what effects the decision would have on other family members. Would one of them be willing to become the caregiver? What community services are available?

Discuss finances, what to do with any existing property, such as the "home place." Is there enough money for an alternate plan to be considered? Who will have power of attorney? Should the primary caregiver have power of attorney? Why or why not? Does everyone feel good about that person having that authority? Don't fail to state any reservations you may have about certain arrangements. Some authorities even say include in the conference those uncooperative members or those who live far away. I think I have mixed feelings about this. Too often the caregiver gets stuck with the care but the far-away siblings want to make financial and placement decisions. Be sure to keep the focus on the current issues—not on past conflicts. Don't be critical of what various members of the family can contribute. Some family members may have conflicts with spouses or work schedules. It is helpful if all the family will at least contribute a cheerful, pleasant attitude and not be disagreeable about everything that is decided upon.

An article in *Parent Care*, "Resources to Assist Family Caregivers," September/October 1989, brings to mind some of the weightier considerations for families on medical decisions—moral and legal dilemmas.

Family caregivers face difficult and often painful times when they make medical treatment decisions for seriously-ill relatives who can no longer choose for themselves. Many feel severe distress, self-doubt, uncertainty, and guilt. Some worry about whether they will make the right decision, be able to carry out their loved one's wishes, or understand the legal issues involved.

Clear specific, up-to-date information is crucial for families who must make decisions for terminally ill relatives. Such a crisis will be easier if the family gathers some information before an emergency arises. Experts from such organizations as the Society for the Right to Die and the U. S. Office of Technology Assessment suggest a number of steps.

1. Discuss the issues. Families member should express their wishes

regarding terminal care as specifically as possible, even though this may be difficult. Relatives who have to guess at their family member's wish may simply make the least guilt-provoking choice or attempt to show their love by demanding that everything possible be done, even if that is contrary to the doctor's advice. Families should also explore whether they feel able to carry out the relative's specific wishes. If family members disagree or do not think they are emotionally capable of complying when the time comes, a person can legally designate someone to act on his/her behalf.

2. Record directives in advance. Written evidence of a patient's wishes offers the best assurance that those desires will be carried out. Most states have living-will laws, and even those states that do not have such statutes consider a living will to be persuasive evidence of the patient's intentions. Living wills declare the patient's directions for medical treatment at the end of life and may also name a proxy or agent, usually a family member, to ensure compliance with these directives.

3. Investigate the legal issues. A living will takes effect only when a patient is diagnosed as terminally ill. Generally, there is no legal difference between withdrawing life-sustaining treatment or withholding it. The courts have held that a person has as much right to stop treatment once it has been started as to reject it in the first place. Furthermore, states that have addressed the issue of withdrawing or withholding nutrition and hydration have determined that artificial feeding (as in nasogastric tubes and intravenous infusion) is a medical treatment that may be rejected. The right to reject it is generally protected by both state and federal constitutions so that patients may exercise the right even if the state's living will act does not permit such rejection.

4. Maximize the chances of compliance. Living wills are not universally recognized across states or within institutional or hospital settings. Since specific legislation varies from state to state, some experts suggest that the best method for maximum protection may be a combination of a living will and a 'durable power of attorney' with the same person being named as proxy in both to ensure that the person appointed can make decisions the patient may not have anticipated.[5]

It is important that a "durable power of attorney" be given to the surrogate decision maker, stating that this power of attorney for health becomes valid upon disability or mental incompetency, otherwise a simple power of attorney (which is usually for finances only) becomes invalid in the event an individual giving this power should become incompetent. An unexpected car accident, a stroke, or an illness resulting in a coma could produce a situation where no one has the proper authority to make valid decisions regarding health care or the implementation of a living will. Discuss with the patient as early as it would seem advisable what kinds of life-sustaining means they would want employed and under what circumstances. Register this with the patient's physician and be sure it is made a part of the patient's chart of his attending physician, as well as the hospital records when the patient is admitted. This relieves the family of any guilt about carrying out the wishes of the patient. The physician has no choice but to follow the wishes expressed. It will be difficult for the caregiver to make the decision, because he is vulnerable to all kinds of pressure and emotions at this time.

Would this "durable power of attorney" raise a question in your mind regarding abuse of privilege by the surrogate decision maker? I am told by my local nursing home ombudsman that a power of attorney can be revoked quite easily should someone get greedy and abusive. One of the responsibilities of the ombudsman is to intercede on behalf of the elderly person, whether he is residing in a nursing home or the home of a caregiver.

The American Association of Retired Persons (AARP) has two free resources that might be helpful to families.

Tomorrow's Choices (D13479) helps families prepare for the unexpected in such areas as finances, living arrangements, and health care.

Health Care Powers of Attorney (D13895) explains this legal document—including a sample form. It is published by the American Bar Association.

These are available from AARP Fulfillment (EE134), 1909 K Street, N. W., Washington, D. C. 20049. Be sure to order by stock number and title.

19

"We've Been There—You, Too, Can Cope"

Nothing gives credence to an argument as does a personal experience or witness. I might try to explain a situation to you but that is just my word. If I bring in a reliable witness who verifies what I have said, my witness becomes more plausible. In the preceding chapters I have bared my heart and soul with you, but it is one person's story. In this chapter I relate the stories of other caregivers, not to try to convince you of the hardships we have had but rather to try to impress on you, the fact that you can make it if this is or will be your lot. You will not be alone, and you will not have been the first to survive it. It is easy for caregivers to get an Elijah complex, feeling that they are the only ones left suffering this way. The truth is there are thousands and thousands who are confronted for the first time with this dilemma. The fact that Dad said on his deathbed, "Promise me you will never put your mother in a nursing home but that you will look after her for me!" overshadows the extenuating situations that may exist later on as we have to consider our spouse, our children, and even our careers.

There is an old proverb or adage, whose source or author I can't recall, that says something like, "I complained that I had no shoes, until I met a man who had no feet." To me, this is a picture of most of us as caregivers. We think no one has ever had it so bad—until we hear another's story. I am indebted to several friends and acquaintances who allowed me to share their stories with you, not to call attention to themselves but that you might be encouraged and, in turn, encourage others who will travel this road.

194

Alice tells her story. When I learned of the hurt and sadness Alice has been through, I was amazed that her genuine happy laughter could ring out so beautifully and echo through my house on that dreary spring morning. I had known a little of the difficulty she had experienced in the care of her mother-in-law and father-in-law but only enough to know I'd like her to share with you.

Alice and her younger brother were placed in a children's home when they were five and three because of the divorce of their parents and their mother's being unable to take care of them. They were in a sense snatched away or kidnapped and deposited several states away in a children's home. Can you imagine the fear these children must have experienced after thinking they were just coming to spend some time with their grandparents and then being thrust into this facility? This is where they grew up, but feelings of distrust were deeply implanted in their minds and, to this day, it is a problem for them to trust people. Alice admits that it might have been the best thing in the world for them because it made them independent, able to stand on their own two feet, and not have to depend on anyone.

Their father's sister Louise, who had no children of her own, often visited these children while they were in the children's home and frequently did things for them. Though Aunt Louise was unable to take them from the home and adopt them, they were with her on holidays and often in the summer. She literally became their surrogate mother and they loved her as such. All the years of their growing up Aunt Louise was the one these children felt closest to. Little wonder then that in the end, Alice and her brother were the ones entrusted with Aunt Louise's care.

Alice married an only child, Tom Jones, who had been adopted by older middle-aged parents when he was five. She had a delightful relationship with her in-laws and they accepted her as their daughter. They shared many happy times, such as when their children were born and they took the newborn infant to the parents' home so Tom's mother could look after everyone (and of course, enjoy the new baby).

It was a good relationship. Alice had in-laws who adored her, and she them. The two families lived next door to each other, and the children hardly knew which house was theirs.

It became almost a weekly ritual with Alice and Mother Jones to go shopping and have lunch, enjoying each other's company. The younger couple were like most of us were at that stage in life so Mother Jones usually treated. Often Mrs. Jones would buy two of whatever she bought so she would have something to share with Alice. By Alice's own admission, few people have as many lovely pieces of silver and crystal as she has because of all the beautiful things she was given. What a delight after growing up not really knowing a mother, to have this generous, loving woman taking such a personal interest in her. They obviously loved each other, and the unyielding lump of distrust slowly began to melt in Alice's heart.

After a long life, Tom's father had a stroke and required much care from the family. From the hospital he had been moved to a nursing home, but he hated it. He would not make an effort to walk to the dining room for his meals, refused the therapy, didn't want to take the medication, and, in general, was very uncooperative. The family urged him to do the things he should so he could be discharged sooner, but he kept saying, "If you will take me home, I promise I will go to the table, eat, and do all the things I am supposed to do." Finally, Alice agreed that they would try it. She knew that the bulk of the care would be upon her since both Mother and Father Jones were elderly by now. He kept his promise and progressed as well as he could. Mother Jones took care of both of them except for the shopping, heavy cleaning, and managing the financial affairs. Her health had remained good.

I believe we all agree that laughter is the best medicine of all. Alice tells the story about one morning very early when Dad Jones called and said, "Come over quick; Mama has gone mute. She can't speak a word." Of course, they dressed and rushed over only to find Mother Jones screaming at him that she had not gone mute but rather that he had gone deaf. He had a temporary hearing loss and as soon as the doctor cleaned his ears, he could hear again. It ended up being a family joke.

After the elder couple had grown older and he had had his stroke, Alice and Tom were given responsibility for the financial end of things by means of a durable power of attorney. The old man never quite trusted Alice, not because of anything she did or any discrepancy but because "she's a woman" and he thought women didn't know about business things. Later he was unhappy because she didn't give him enough money. She and Tom learned that the money was never spent but was placed in his wallet in his handkerchief drawer. It became an easy thing to "recirculate" twenty dollars of the money and Daddy Jones never knew the difference since he never counted it or spent it.

When Alice would show him how she had managed his funds and how well he was doing with her management, he would be pleased, but something in him kept him from believing a woman could be that smart.

Daddy Jones died in his eighties and that left Mother Jones alone in the house. This seemed to work well enough for awhile, but when Tom's career took him to another state, Mother Jones had to come with them since she had no one else to look after her. It was at this time that she moved in with the younger Joneses and their children. What a chore to combine two households with two women loving their possessions and not wanting to part with a single thing. They somehow accomplished it and kept their relationship intact because they loved each other. Alice says she never heard Mother Jones say an unkind or negative word about anyone. To this day, she can't fault her about anything—except growing old, as if that were possible to prevent.

Having an elderly person underfoot all day and all night with teenagers in the house soon began to wear on Alice's nerves. The children began to want to be somewhere else but home, because "Grandma is always around." The family had moved to a large house in a rural area, but Tom's profession took him into town every day and most nights. His work also involved Alice much of the time, so having a sitter became a problem and they were fearful of leaving Mother Jones alone. Her mind was not as clear as it once was. She began to wander off. In other words, she could not be left alone anymore, and Alice was realizing she had to make a decision about being a full-time mother to teenagers or be a full-time caregiver to Mother Jones. Alice and Tom decided that the children and the younger family unit had to come first. It was evident that Alice could not physically or emotionally do both.

Tom and Alice did a thorough investigation of the options open to them. Now they faced the difficult part of committing Mother Jones. A trip was coming up that would take Alice away for several days. This seemed like the time to make the break. One day Alice just drove Mother Jones over to a mini-home where four other elderly residents lived in a private home and told her that she was going to stay there for awhile. They had to make a trip and she could not stay by herself.

I asked Alice about the response from Mother Jones. She did not become emotional or cry. Nor did she make accusations or say hurtful things. This was a very painful thing for Alice and she ached for having to do it. She says she is glad that she admitted her alone because it would have been very difficult on Tom. The situation was not made any easier by the talk going around at their church criticizing Alice for not keeping Mrs. Jones in the home. It is so much easier to criticize when one is on the outside looking in. Those who criticize so freely are the ones that suppose since there were no preschool or small children in the house, there was no reason why Alice couldn't keep Mrs. Jones. It was the least she could do after all the elder Joneses had done for them.

Mrs. Jones never asked to come home and never fussed about the home except to say that the administrator was mean. Frequent visits were made and Mother Jones was taken home for special occasions but once she was settled in the mini-home, it became home to her.

Later it fell Alice's lot to help care for her Aunt Louise, who had been so wonderful and loving to her and her brother. She lived

200 miles away, so seeing her frequently was hard to do. When Alice did visit, she tried to stay a couple of days and do those things that would cheer her up.

Alice would take her shopping for new gowns and shoes, take her to lunch at a favorite place, or drive past the new subdivisions or other places in the city that might interest her. The distance and the infrenquency of visits did not diminish the feeling of responsibility Alice had. In her later years, Aunt Louise became an expert at making one feel guilty. She retained her mental faculties and once, when Alice visited, Aunt Louise wanted to be taken to look for a new nursing home because she didn't like the way things were going where she was. They did and she asked to be moved.

Part of that time Alice had the responsibility for two older ladies, plus high school- and college-age children. Alice confided that she feels church friends don't really understand and support families going through these trying times. If she had it to do over, she doesn't feel she would do things very differently today. As she said, "We did the best we could at the time with all the other things going on in our lives. What we did we did in love—not just for a parent and an aunt, but for our children as well."

During this later time, things were not going too well with Tom's job and he ultimately accepted an invitation to join another organization; so another move and more trauma.

Alice has made a valid observation for all of us. She feels that friends and acquaintances don't sympathize and grieve as they should with families whose loved ones die in nursing homes. It is as if some think the grieving is over and that the separation and death really occurred much earlier. She also says that too few realized her loss when her aunt died because they did not know of the close relationship that existed there.

My friend Mary would say that trouble always seems to come in pairs. When you know her situation, you will agree.

"Being an only child makes it doubly hard on a family when an elderly person is in the home to be cared for. When I was growing up and during my younger adult days, Mother and I were very close and enjoyed each other, but that situation is deteriorating now. I am having real trouble with my anger. I have to keep remembering that Mother is not the same anymore and in a sense not responsible.

"My mother was (and is) a very independent woman who lived in her own home until she was ninety-two. Quite a feat, wouldn't you say? During that time she rented out her spare bedroom and that gave her someone in the house and a sense of security. She was mentally alert and managed her own affairs until she had a stroke and could not live alone any longer.

"It was quite a hassle getting her to move in with us five years ago but we felt we had no alternative. I surely couldn't go over there and live with her. It just seemed best that she live with us. (From time to time I also had my mother-in-law living with us, but not on a regular basis. At the time I thought it worked out as well as it could. I was not completely tied down at that time.)

"Of course, you know what it is to try to impress a ninety-two-year-old that she must get rid of most of her household things. That in itself was an ordeal since to her that meant the end of independence. We moved her in upstairs but my house is one of those not arranged well for invalid or semi-invalid persons to get around in. I was constantly worried about her falling down the steps. Eventually, she deteriorated to the point that she could not manage the steps; therefore, in the last few months we have moved her downstairs in the living room on a hospital bed. At least now she is on the same floor with me and my husband and also close to a bathroom, but we have a portable potty by the bed also.

"You know I have always been involved at my own church and in church work throughout the area, and I miss that so much now."

Let me tell you something about Mary. Mary has always been a warm, interesting, vivacious, outgoing person with a wonderful sense of humor and laughter. She says to be home all the time and to have to give up all outside activity has worked a real hardship on her, even to the point of her becoming angry and resentful. To get to church on a Sunday morning now is a real treat. She can no longer get there to teach a class or play the piano or be involved in any way other than just to put in an appearance.

"I know it is risky, but on Sunday I turn on the television, prop Mother up in bed, pull up the rails of the bed, explain to her where I am going, and slip out for at least part of the service. You know I live so close to the church I can be home in a minute. After taking care of everything I am so tired that I find it difficult to even stay awake sometimes. As soon as the service is over, I fly back home not really knowing what I will find. Recently, Mother had managed to get up and had turned the potty over making a great mess in the living room.

"Mother is a very demanding woman and insists that things have to be done her way. She has developed some 'quirky' little habits and ideas, such as, thinking she has to have the window in her bedroom open each night regardless of the outside temperature. If it is raining, then the air conditioner has to be on, thereby freezing everyone else to death. Since she is still somewhat mobile, she gets up and turns things on after they have been turned off. This is especially a problem when my mother-in-law is here because she nearly freezes. Mother is constantly wanting her clothes rearranged or taken off, or sleeves rolled up or down. There isn't a consistent pattern but it got so bad a few weeks ago I asked the doctor to give her some medication so she wouldn't be so restless. I feel a lot of it is a part of the ploy to get attention. I have to keep reminding myself that I am dealing with a ninety-seven-year-old child who is accustomed to having her way. Frankly, I am having a hard time dealing with my anger about Mother's behavior.

"One of the things that gets next to me most and hurts so is Mother's yelling at me and ordering me around. When I am preparing dinner and come into the living room to sit down a minute, she will yell in her grating little voice, 'You're just sitting there! When you gonna fix my supper? I'm hungry.' At about 11:00 in the morning she will start saying, 'Fix my lunch! Fix my lunch! I want my lunch now!'

"When it appears that I am really involved in something or with someone and not where she can see me, she begins saying, 'I need to potty—whoever you are talking to will have to wait. Stop what you are doing and come help me use the potty or I'll wet the bed.'"

Mary's mother has learned that she can dominate and control Mary by demanding things and threatening the consequences if Mary doesn't obey. Mary says that for some time now she has been unable to reason anything with her mother. It appears that when she makes up her mind about something, that is the way it is going to be.

She has to get up to go to the bathroom three and four times a night; therefore, when the night is over, poor Mary feels as if she has had no sleep at all. Mary is amazed at how often her mother has to urinate. In exasperation, one day Mary said, "Mother, you must be made of urine—and you don't drink that much."

Mary's mother has little use of her right side since her stroke, but she insists on eating by herself with her left hand (she is right-handed). Getting her into the wheelchair and to the table is difficult enough, but after she eats, she is in such a mess she has to be stripped and bathed. Even the plastic bibs don't protect her adequately. Of course, the floor then needs to be cleaned.

Since her Mother's last stroke, Mary has to do all those personal things for her mother, even taking care of all the bathroom necessities. Mary's mother is a small woman fortunately, so Mary can manage to get her in the bathtub. She has a bath bench to sit her on, but she is so tottery she must be supported all the time to keep her from falling.

Sadly, Mary laments the fact that her mother is not like she used to be. Whereas she was once very independent, she is now very possessive, demanding, impatient, and unreasonable. It has been very hard for Mary to keep up with her housework, laundry, cooking, and take care of two older ladies.

Mary's mother-in-law, who is only eighty-three, is an entirely different person. She will only ask for something if there is no way she can get it for herself. Her mother-in-law has helped out in the past, but now she has had several strokes, by-pass surgery, a pacemaker installed, and heart failures. She is in a rehabilitation center herself. When she leaves this facility, she will probably come to Mary and John's home once again. Fortunately, her different personality will be much less demanding.

About two years ago the doctor told Mary that her mother probably couldn't live more than six weeks and suggested she call a hospice. The hospice staff came and ministered for six months—her mother is still living. Mary put her in a nursing home for a few months, but it was eating up her little savings at the rate of $2,000 a month and Mary was fearful they wouldn't have enough to bury her. I advised her to check with Medicaid to see what help was available.

The pattern is so predictable. Is it any wonder that Mary and John find themselves snapping at each other? They both knew they needed some time together but finding help was so hard and money was not too plentiful.

"I was completely fatigued and nothing I did was right. There was never a private moment with my husband. I have had to drop out of everything that I enjoyed doing, and I just told my husband I could not take it anymore. Fortunately, we were given a gift certificate for a few days at the hotel, and that has helped so much. I don't believe I could have made it without some sort of help.

"My daughter made a suggestion that I have been trying to follow. She said, 'Mom, why don't you try to look at Grandma as if she were Jesus.' I have tried that and it does help some but my mind always seems to go back to 'but Jesus wouldn't act the way she does.' I am working on that but it is hard. I often wonder if I had tried to apply that from the beginning, would it have helped."

Up until now, Mary and John have been using their own funds for her mother's expenses. I urged her to check with her lawyer about using her mother's money. She has a durable power of attorney and there are no siblings, but Mary seems to have an aversion to doing this. Families can get in deep financial trouble when they take on the financial responsibility of an elderly loved one.

Mary says the secret of her being able to hang on this long is the love of her family and the prayers of her church people. I have a Christian friend who says that people who say they are praying for you should put feet on those prayers and instead of praying so much, should come to the house and spend the afternoon with a shut-in and give the caregiver a few hours' help. She makes a good point!

Laura is an attractive, young, middle-age professional woman who seems to a have an unusually heavy load at this time in her life. She is the only child of parents who married later in life and doted on her.

Her father's profession made it possible for the family to enjoy many of the comforts of life and for this she is very grateful. It was a happy home and having a good relationship with her parents as she was growing up makes it easier to carry the burden of her parents' illnesses now.

Laura married Gary when they were teenagers. She reports that her parents helped them in every conceivable way. The thought has occurred to her that maybe less indulgence would have been better for the marriage and for them individually, but it seemed to be a good marriage for many years. Unfortunately, now they are going through a very painful divorce. There are children in the family, but Laura feels hesitant to share things with her children because of appearing to be putting them in the middle, so she largely is carrying her load alone.

For as long as Laura can remember her mother has been ill, to one degree or another, getting better for awhile and being able to take care of the home and family, but never really a healthy person. Growing up with her mother being sick so much made Laura mature earlier. As a young person she often did things her mother ordinarily would have done. Her mother's health has deteriorated with age. She has had numerous surgeries and hospital stays. With this background, it is easy to see how Laura became a caregiver early in life. Looking back now, she realizes she became an adult early, making adult decisions. She never really felt "put-upon" as a child but only regretful that her mother frequently was ill.

Her parent's whole life revolved around her and at times it was somewhat smothering but not really in an oppressive way. It has remained so throughout her adult life as well.

Her mother is a dominant person, and if they had lived nearby it might have caused a great deal of trouble.

Since her parents do live so far away, Laura does a lot of caregiving via long distance. This situation is very hard on the caregiver. It is difficult to find live-in help and very discouraging to the child when the aging parents constantly fire the help.

Through the years Laura's father has been able physically to assist her mother, but several months ago he was told that he has a terminal illness. Both parents are strong willed but are coping well. Yet at times they refuse to deal with the reality of a terminal illness. Laura helps keep them focused and is an encourager to them, promoting the concept "one day at a time."

Families caring for families is not new to Laura because as a child she remembers that her father cared for her grandfather. Her father did have a brother, but he refused to share in the caregiving. As so often is the case, the one who has no part of the caregiving always questions how the money is being spent and issues all sorts of unreasonable demands when the father dies. Seeing her parents care for her grandfather and later her uncle gave Laura a wonderful role model.

When Laura was in high school, her father also cared for another brother who had a malignancy and was not covered by insurance. So caregiving is sort of second nature because of her parent's role in taking care of family members.

Laura's caregiving has consisted largely of helping her parents make decisions about their future. They are both mentally competent so she does not make decisions for them; rather she gives them her opinions and research, helping them make the decisions they can live with. She is eager for them to continue taking care of their own business as long as possible; but when they can no longer do this, they have arranged (legally) for Laura to do it for them.

There is no resentment in Laura's heart about the care of her parents—they have always done so much for her and her family. They have looked upon her husband as their own son and have treated him as such—even to the point of educating him. One of Laura's hurts now is his rejection of them. Fortunately, her parents are financially independent and this especially is a blessing since she is going through a divorce and she doesn't have to worry about personally being able to care for them financially. She never questions or thinks about whether it is her place to care for them now. She feels she has a good healthy relationship with them, but since they are financially independent, she wants them to continue to make decisions knowing she is there to assist or affirm them.

An interesting aspect of Laura's case is how the roles have suddenly been reversed since she told them of her impending divorce. Whereas, before they seemed to lean on her heavily, now at this point they are trying to be the strong ones, not wanting to put anything else on her, even to the point of making light of their own ailments so she won't worry. In a strange turn of events, Laura thinks this may be good for them. But since she confers often with the doctors, she knows the truth of their situation.

Through the years Laura has gradually become her parents' protector, shielding them from all the hurts and disappointments she was going through. A case in point is the news of her divorce, which she did not share with them for some time though she really needed their love, comfort, and support. She did not want to add to their burden of poor health. Finally, she had to share her hurt with them because she was not strong enough to carry this by herself. They responded first with denial, then blaming themselves or saying surely something could be worked out. She had been so guarded and stoic until now that they were unprepared for her emotional release of tears. They cried too—they were heartsick. At their age, they are unaccustomed to the idea of a divorce in their family. She is their little girl again and they are making every effort to "make it right—make it not hurt anymore." For them to become her protector again temporarily gave some relief to her in carrying such a heavy load. Up until this time of agony in her marriage, she had assumed the parent role for a long time but now it had reversed again.

Laura's load has also been made heavier by trying to keep details of her own life from her children.

One of the ways that she has offered care is in helping her parents find other doctors, maybe for a second opinion rather than just settling for hometown advice. By reminding them of some of the things they used to tell her about taking care of herself, she has been able to convince them of the value of seeking out other opinions. She did the research, she knew the questions to ask, how to make arrangements and accomplish what they finally agreed to. This was accomplished medically and even the doctors say her father's living this long is a miracle. Laura attributes this amazing feat to his strong will to live to be able to see her through this hard time, plus his strong faith in Christ. He has already outlived his doctor's predictions. It was also a relief to Laura to find that her parents have both made living wills, sparing her the possible trauma of having to make a hard decision about their medical treatment. (See chapter 20 for a discussion of living wills.)

There is a double load here because her mother is facing another surgery. She has already had multiple surgeries and is a poor candidate because of her heart condition. The surgery added to the stresses this caregiver already has. Laura is an only child; she lives far away from her sick parents; she has her own profession to try to hold together; she had to move from her lovely home; her marriage has broken up and she faces the uncertain future alone; she is dealing with a feeling of rejection and bitterness; she has deliberately distanced herself from her children so as not to make them feel as if they must choose sides; and she has the sole care of two elderly people, one of whom is terminally ill. How alone can one person be? The type of care that will be required for the surviving parent is another concern that must be faced down the road at some point.

Here is another caregiver's story with a little different slant. As I share this one, you might ask, How can three women let their only brother take care of the personal needs of their mother in her demented infirmed old age? Apparently, it is easy; just look the other way, don't come around, and be sure you don't call and ask if you can do anything.

Bill was the child who stayed near his parents through the years, living not too far away. As the parents grew older, he was the one who pitched in and helped his dad with home and farm chores, plus carrying on his own profession. It seemed like no big deal for years as the two men enjoyed each other and working together gave them time alone as father and son.

When Bill's mother became ill and needed help, the girls were always too busy with their own families or careers. Bill's wife had never had a good relationship with her in-laws because they were critical of her language and habits.

Before long, Bill's father had grown so feeble he could not care for the farm or even for his wife, and good help was not available. But the older couple would not even discuss selling the farm. The older man kept insisting that he would soon be better and could continue as he had been doing for years. He would not even agree that the cattle could be sold.

Domestic help and nursing care that was available was expensive, and again the older couple insisted they did not need to spend that money on help. Bill knew better. The farm looked like a jungle and the house didn't resemble in the least the way his mother used to keep it. His own job kept him from taking over the farm and care of his parents.

Bill tried to call a family conference, but one sister said she lived too far away, another said her career took precedence, and the other was going through a divorce and she was having to seek employment to provide for herself and her children; but all of them stated unequivocally they were not in favor of putting mother and dad in a nursing home. Bill's wife said the old folks should have thought about how it would be when they got old and needed someone when they were so cruel in their criticism of her. Sorry, count her out, too.

Bill would go over each morning and evening and do as much for his parents as he could. He found some workers for the farm, but instead of helping, the farm was pulling the family fast into bankruptcy. With the help of a lawyer, Bill finally convinced his still mentally competent father that they must sell off part of the farm for living expenses, because Bill could not manage his own job and take care of the farm and them, too. This infuriated the sisters because selling the farm meant the loss of part of their inheritance. It was the thing that alienated the whole family—even Bill's wife didn't think it was the thing to do. She thought they could have "outlasted" the old folks and that would have been a nice little nest egg for them and their children. Bill finally got his father to agree to giving him power of attorney. This further infuriated the sisters.

Bill's father voluntarily went to an old veteran's home and lived out his remaining years away from his family. He was placed in a nursing home for awhile but the money was fast giving out and he knew there would be nothing left to take care of Mama. He felt this was his only option.

For years each morning, Bill would go over and bathe and feed his mother, who had dementia and knew practically nothing. At first it was very difficult for him to do this but since there was no one else, he did it. Sitters who helped out did just that—sit. How sad! His parents each died away from the other; the children are estranged; and Bill is married to an unforgiving and unbending wife. He and Job in the Old Testament have at least that one thing in common.

What hurt and anger can be caused over a piece of land that will still be here and belong to someone else long after family members are gone.

20

Who or What Is Out There to Help Me?

As I look back over our experience with Ted's parents, I wonder how many good things were out there that I did not know existed. How much could they have helped us? Why didn't someone tell us? Did they exist at that time?

One of the things I hope to accomplish with this book is to make you, the reader, aware of the possibilities of help to see you through. I could not possibly name them all, and services differ from state to state. Hopefully, however, you will get an idea of how to begin seeking out what will help you most.

Services for elderly persons in the community are increasing across our country. Under the Older Americans Act, each state has established an office on aging. Most states have designated area agencies on aging to serve older people in specific communities. The very best place to begin to find out what is available and who is eligible is to contact your local Area Agency on Aging. Every state has an Area Agency on Aging (AAA), a governmental source or channel for all federal and some private programs for senior adults. All federal funds are channeled through AAA. This agency is one way to get into various programs for information and help.

A word about the Older Americans Act might be helpful. This information that I share came from a report of the Special Committee on Aging, United States Senate, 1987.

The Older Americans Act carried a broad mandate to improve the lives of older persons in the areas of income, emotional and physical well-being, housing, employment, social services, civic, cultural, and recreational opportunities.

The purpose of Title III of the Act, which authorizes formula grants to states for services to older persons, is to foster the development of a comprehensive and coordinated service system for older persons in order to: (a) Secure and maintain maximum independence and dignity in a home environment for older persons capable of self-care; (b) remove individual and social barriers to economic and personal independence for older persons; and (c) provide a continuum of care for the vulnerable elderly.

Under Title III, grants are made to state agencies on aging, which in turn award funds to 670 area agencies on aging, to plan, coordinate, and advocate for a comprehensive service system for older persons. Title III supports a wide range of supportive services, as well as congregate and home-delivered nutrition services. Certain supportive services have been given priority by Congress. These priority services are access services (transportation, outreach, information and referral), legal assistance, and in-home services such as homemaker, home health aide, personal care, chore, escort and shopping services. Visiting and telephone reassurance are also considered to be in-home supportive services. Other community-based long-term care services which may be provided under Title III include case management, adult day care, and respite care.

The Older Americans Act Amendments of 1987 (Public Law 100-175), which authorized the Act for another 4 years, created a new service program for in-home services for the frail elderly.[1]

Many programs such as Home Care, Meals-on-Wheels, Alzheimer's support groups, Helping Hand, Respite programs, Home Health Care, and many other services are contracted out by the Area Agency on Aging and are to help older Americans maintain independence and dignity at home and to prevent unnecessary nursing-home admissions.

In rural areas the county senior-citizens center is another good source of information. In my community, the nursing-home ombudsman is located in the senior-citizens center in quarters provided by AAA, though the program itself is sponsored largely by the United Way. This ombudsman is the one to talk to regarding any nursing-home problems or even abuse of the elderly in a private home. It is important that families know they can complain about things that are not right in a nursing home. This is the work of the ombudsman. It is against the law to kick out residents who complain. In most of the better- staffed senior-citizens centers we find health model day-care centers, operating financially on a sliding scale, with nurses and physical therapists on duty all day. As these health model day-care centers are becoming more available, they are alternatives to a regular nursing home. They will take all kinds of persons who need this kind of medical assistance and daily care. Of course, it is a day program only.

We also find social model day-care centers with no medical or nurse assistance, but a person must be continent and able to do a number of things for himself. This program is geared toward activities and life fulfillment. Part of this group might tend a garden, be involved in crafts, or any number of other things.

At a multipurpose senior-citizens center numerous activities are going on all the time. I believe all the centers are nutrition sites for balanced, hot meals; in addition to this, meals are sent out over the community on a daily basis. Shelf meals are also provided to shut-ins in the event weather or something else should prevent the volunteers from the delivery. This is not the same as Meals-on-Wheels, though it is located in the same complex in our city.

The senior-citizens center also offers classes in Spanish, oil painting, crafts of all kinds, exercise, square dancing, and even gardening. There are also classes on nutrition and other health-related subjects. The American Association of Retired Persons (AARP) has volunteers who will assist in filling out medical forms for Medicare/ Medicaid (as will the social worker). Near tax-filing time, AARP also provides assistance in completing income-tax forms. On a regular basis, blood pressure is taken and cholesterol measured—free of charge for those over sixty-five. In addition, there are many things available which I have not enumerated.

Another source of possible assistance is Home Health-Care Services. This service provides support services for many hospital-discharged patients who need some assistance but who do not want to enter a nursing home or to live with their children. It would behoove children of elderly parents to check out all possibilities for assistance before taking on the responsibility for the total care of their parent. This would reduce the stress level in the life of the caregiving child; it would help the elderly retain a sense of independence and thus avoid or delay giving up control of their lives as long as possible; and it would relieve the parent of possible guilt feelings because of having to live with a child. In the past, an illness that involved hospitalization usually meant a stint in a skilled-care nursing home or some other health-related facility before being able to return to one's own home.

James Halpern, in his book *Helping Your Aging Parents* suggests that a hospital discharge planner will assist a patient in formulating a plan to care for needs. The family should be involved in these decisions and should know in advance how much these services will cost.[2]

Home-care agencies offer the services of registered nurses, licensed practical nurses, physical therapists and their assistants, social workers, homemakers, and home health aides. The home health aide is also called a personal-care service worker. These assist a disabled person to function within her own home. There are three levels of care provided:

1. Provides assistance with the care of the environment, including such tasks as dusting, cleaning, and cooking.
2. Provides personal care—bathing, dressing, and the like—as well as assistance with the environment.
3. Provides level 1 and level 2 care plus assistance with the administration of medication, changing of dressings, and so forth.[3]

Support groups are another way to seek help for ourselves or for our loved ones. It is very advantageous for us as caregivers and for the patient to seek out those persons who truly know what we are experiencing. In these groups we can "let our hair down" and tell it as it is. In all probability there will be someone there who has been through the same kinds of things. In these groups it is all right to say you hate your situation or you are mad at your husband, children, or siblings for their seeming unconcerned attitude about the disabled person. It is a place where you don't have to put on a front. If you want to weep that is OK, too. Here you can take off the mask and reveal your true feelings about your situation. You will get a sympathetic ear. The group relationships give you the opportunity to relate happenings as well as ask for opinions or what you might expect next or how the group would have reacted or responded in the same situation. Most of us are glad to share ways we have managed in various circumstances. These groups may be specifically organized, such as for caregivers of Alzheimer's victims. They might be groups of friends or church members. Sometimes the more highly organized groups may have a speaker who is helpful. Just to be able to ask questions or say exactly how we feel, as unflattering as it might be, without feeling condemned is a real release.

Fortunately, support groups are not just for the caregiver but also for victims of diseases. A friend had a mastectomy. Before she left the hospital, a member of a support group called on her and urged her to join their group for her own help but also to learn what she could do for others. Some of the groups, such as the Alzheimer's, will even provide a sitter for the caregiver so that she can get away for a few hours.

The greatest support networks we find are those relationships in our churches, communities, immediate neighborhoods, among our co-workers, and in our civic organizations. When an older person leaves his job, his church, and his familiar neighborhood, it is a real blow to his support network. A family has to weigh very carefully the advisability of moving a parent out of even a deteriorating neighborhood against the emotional losses of this familiar support system. In these older neighborhoods, it is common for neighbors to linger over fences or drop in periodically just to talk and check on one another. Many hot loaves of bread or plates of cookies have been exchanged over the years. These relationships are like the glue that holds our self-esteem together.

Support of the elderly from their own families is so important. I have often thought how "interesting" that at the time in our lives when we are most vulnerable and prone to be ill, without financial resources, looking old, unable physically to do everything we want to, we have the most trauma in our lives, including the probable loss of a spouse and being moved from the home we have know and loved for years. Most of us are very ready to give advice about what our parent(s) should do about various things—and that is appreciated. But from what I've read and from what my in-laws said, it is far more important to write, call, or spend time with them. To be old, widowed, alone, and many times ill is almost more than one can bear. As persons grow older, their need for touching, hugging, and contact in general does not diminish but rather increases. At this time physical contact is very important. A widow told my husband, "The thing I think I miss most is being held and hugged every day."

In our city there is a model social organization called the Helping Hand. It is made up of volunteers who go into the homes of caregivers for respite purposes. Many of these volunteers have had experience in caring for patients with dementia. I understand many other areas of the country are modeling an organization after this one. These volunteers are trained in seminars and are usually sent out the first few times with an experienced worker. If this type of service is needed, the caregiver should call the Alzheimer's Disease and Related Disorders Association for further information. It is amazing what two hours out of the house can do for a person who feels she has reached the breaking point.

If your senior-citizens center is a multipurpose program, call to see if they have Health Day-Care and what the conditions and rates per day are. The change will likely do the patient good and you can rest assured of her care. Since every community and state differs, it is difficult to be too definitive but it takes only a minute to call the center or the Area Agency on Aging. Be sure to make notes and get names of persons you talk to so that when you call again you can ask for the same person and not have to repeat everything.

The hospice concept evolved from homes established centuries ago by religious orders to provide personal attention and care for the sick and dying poor. The first hospice program in the United State was started in 1971 in Connecticut. The movement has now grown to more than 1,500 programs over the country.[4] Hospice is an alternative for the terminally ill person who does not want to die in a hospital or other medical facility. Most hospice patients do die in their own homes with their family around. Hospice is a system of care for dying patients and their families. About 90 percent of the patients served by these programs are cancer patients. The focus in hospice, according to Halpern, "is not on seeking a cure but on caring for patients and supporting both patients and their families with respect to a variety of needs."[5] The hospice idea is that patients should be allowed to die with dignity, without life-support measures being employed or any heroic measures taken. Hospice staff also work to see that the patient has a death as pain free as possible. The hospice works with the family to try to make the remaining days peaceful and meaningful. The family members care for the patient with regular visits from the physician, nurses, social workers, home health aides, and other hospice staff as required by the family. The fact that the patient is going to die has been accepted by hospice team members and the family; therefore, all are involved with the patient in the dying process. The aim of the hospice is not only to assist the patient in dying but also to prepare and strengthen the family for the coming death of a loved one. Most hospices also have a clergyman on staff to assist the family in the grieving process.

Care is given, by and large, in the patient's home. There are some hospice agencies located in nursing homes or hospitals, but most have a home focus and are community based. Different localities have hospice agencies and can be reached through most of the channels discussed earlier.

The philosophy of hospice and the nursing home is totally different. The nursing-home focus has been maintenance and custodial care in an environment which has become the residence of the patient. I am afraid many nursing homes while trying to prolong life are destroying the reason and will to live of the patients by ignoring the same basic philosophies found in the hospice principles. In contrast, within the hospice concept death is the plan of care for the terminally ill.

Hospice costs are usually much lower than hospitals or nursing homes because neither room and board nor life-support systems have to be paid for. The federal government has realized that hospice is an alternative to regular hospital care, so if certain provisions are met, Medicare will pay for it. The negative part of this is Medicare certification. Only a small percentage of hospices take part in the Medicare programs because of the stringent regulations.[6] Even if payment must be made from the family's funds, the fees are based on a sliding scale and are usually very reasonable.

If you have questions about hospice care that you can't get answered locally, try calling Hospicelink, a toll-free, national information service. The number is 1-800-331-1620. (In Connecticut or Alaska, call 203/767-1620.) Hospicelink is a nonprofit group based in Essex, Connecticut, and is not affiliated with any particular hospice but is a part of the Hospice Education Institute.

Meals-on-Wheels (or home-delivered meals) is another option for persons who live alone and are not physically able to prepare meals for themselves. These are either totally subsidized or are on a sliding scale, determined by the income of the person who is over sixty-five.

My daughter-in-law's grandmother is a spunky, little woman with all her mental faculties who is determined that she is not going into a long-term care facility or live with any of her children.

So she lives alone with a little device called Lifeline that allows her assisted independence.

According to Art Linkletter's book *Old Age Is Not for Sissies*, Lifeline is now being used by more than one hundred thousand people in the United States and Canada and the number is growing. The system offers security and help at the touch of a waterproof button that be can worn even in the shower.

Senior citizens who are alone, disabled, frail, or recovering from an illness or surgery, can subscribe to this service for a small fee per month. It is backed up by twenty-four-a-day emergency help. The program links the subscribers to a hospital emergency room and directly to the Lifeline Center in Massachusetts. A small wireless button is worn on a slender chain around the neck. When the button is pressed, a radio signal is sent. The system works even if the phone is off the hook or if there has been a power failure. If a subscriber loses consciousness during a medical emergency, a timer automatically continues to signal for help.[7]

A free publication that came with my local newspaper at the beginning of the year gives a complete listing of all the services and agencies in our area related to senior citizens, both priced and free. It gives a brief description of the service, eligibility requirements, telephone numbers and office hours, plus whom to contact for more information. If your area does not have such a publication, it would be a great project for senior citizens to work on getting put together and published. This one was sponsored in part by Humana Hospital, Lexington; Lexington-Fayette Urban County Government; Mayor's Office on Aging; and Lexington Senior Citizens Center. This one is entitled *Information for Older Adults*.

Should you like to have information about the living will, this may be obtained by writing The Society for the Right to Die, 250 W. 57th Street, New York, New York 10107.

Conclusion

When I began this book, I stated in the introduction that it is not conclusive nor is it a medical journal. It is just one caregiver telling another how she tried to cope and where she found sustenance.

There have been days as I was writing that I dreaded to get to work because I knew of the emotional drain it would cause. So many of the feelings that I had filed away in the archives of my mind had to be brought back out in the light to be reviewed, re-thought, worked through, cried over, grieved with, and suffered in. In a way, it has been a catharsis. I still blush with guilt at some of the feelings I had then, but the overriding feeling is one of joy and enrichment.

I have come to stand in awe at the human mind and the many intricacies of it. Oh, how complex is all of life! I am reminded of the Scripture that says, "Who hath known the mind of the Lord?" (Rom. 11:34, KJV). How wonderfully and fearfully we are made! (See Ps. 139:14).

Now that I have reached the completion of this book, after I have read the story of many other caregivers, I know how blessed I was to have such wonderful in-laws. I wish that I might be the kind of in-law that I had in my father-in-law and mother-in-law. They were the epitome of what in-laws should be. They made me feel that I was their first choice for their son's wife. They never failed to receive the help I offered with anything other than a profound sense of gratitude. There is a lovely poem whose author is unknown that says in part what I feel for my mother and father-in-law.

Touching Shoulders

. . . It is just a sweet memory that chants the refrain:
"I'm glad I touched shoulders with you!"
Did you know you were brave, did you know you were strong?
Did you know there was one leaning hard?
Did you know that I waited and listened and prayed,
And was cheered by your simplest word?
Did you know that I longed for that smile on your face,
For the sound of your voice ringing true?
Did you know I grew stronger and better because
I had merely touched shoulders with you?
I am glad that I live, that I battle and strive
For the place that I know I must fill;
I am thankful for sorrows; I'll meet with a grin
What fortune may send, good or ill.
I may not have wealth, I may not be great,
But I know I shall always be true,
For I have in my life that courage you gave
When once I rubbed shoulders with you.[1]

Notes

Chapter 3

1. *The Atlanta Constitution*, "Plastic Masks Aid to Cancer Patients," Friday, Aug. 19, 1977, Sec. 18-A.

Chapter 9

1. "Outer Space" by Theodore Sisk, Copyright 1969 by Sylena Music Co. International copyright secured. All rights reserved.

Chapter 14

1. Mildred Wade, "A Letter to My Mother," copyright 1985. All rights reserved. Used by permission of the author.

Chapter 15

1. Marjorie George, *Aide Magazine*, USAA, San Antonio, TX, Dec. 1989, "Who Will Help You When You Help Your Parents?", 15.
2. Jean Maxwell, *Centers for Older People, N. Y.: The National Council on Aging*, 1962 as part of "Ten Basic Concepts of Aging." Resource files from office of Bluegrass LTC Ombudsman.
3. Ruth Kay, *Plain Talk About Aging*, NIMH, Ky. Division of Mental Health, Cabinet for Human Resources Publications Library, Lexington, Ky. DHHS Pub. # (ADM) 83-1266, GPO:1983 O-412-919: QL3.
4. *Developments in Aging: 1987*, Vol. 3, "The Long-Term Care Challenge", US Govn. Printing Office, Washington, DC: 1988, 5-10.
5. Pamphlet: *A Profile of Older Americans*: 1989, Program Resources Dept., AARP, AoA, US Dept. HHS, 1, para. 6.
6. Ibid.
7. Ibid: AARP Pamphlet, 3-4
8. Ibid.
9. Royal H. Roussel, *Aging: Special Issue on Independence,* US DHHS, #349 1985, "Aging Upward: How to Win While Growing Old," 19-22.
10. Robert Browning, *Rabbi Ben Ezra*, "Masterpieces of Religious Verse", edited by James Dalton Morrison (Harper & Row, NY and Evanston, 1948), 77, #239.

Chapter 16

1. Partial information gleaned from the following ADRDA topical brochures. Reprinted with permission from Alzheimer's Disease and Related Disorders Association.
—Alzheimer's Disease and Related Disorders: A description of the dementias.
—Alzheimer's Disease: An Overview
—When the Diagnosis Is Alzheimer's
—Memory and Aging
—Alzheimer's Newsletter, Spring and Summer, 1989
2. Ibid: ADRDA.
3. Ibid: ADRDA.
4. Ibid: ADRDA.

5. *Lexington Herald Leader*, AP, May 8, 1990, "Study Finds Gene that May Be Linked to Alzheimer's Disease."

6. Dina Van Pelt, *Insight Magazine*, March 1989, "Nose May Be First Site of Alzheimer's," 58.

7. *Lexington Herald Leader*, Sec. A-3, May 4, 1990, "Brain Tissue Grows in Laboratory Dish."

8. Nancy Mace and Peter Rabins, "The 36-Hour Day," *The Johns Hopkins University Press*, 1981, 130.

9. Ibid. Ch. 7.

10. Tom Whatson, *Christian Herald*, October 1988, "Stronger Than Alzheimer's."

(Much of the information in this chapter has been gleaned from the library and resource files of the office of the Bluegrass LTC Ombudsman, Lexington, Ky.).

Chapter 17

1. Nancy Fox, *you, your parent, and the nursing home*, "The Family Guide to Long-Term Care," Geriatric Press, Inc. 1982, Ch. 2, 31.

2. *The Ombudsman Connection*, Vol. 6, #1, Spring 1990, Lexington, Kentucky

3. Op.cit., Fox, 33-44.

4. *Louisville Courier Journal*, Louisville, Ky., Series in May 1980.

5. Art Linkletter, *Old Age Is Not For Sissies*(Penguin Books 1989), 141.

6. *Developments in Aging: 1987*, Vol. 3, "The Long-Term Care Challenge", A Report of the Special Committee on Aging, US Senate, Pursuant to S.Res. 80, Sec.19, January 28, 1987. Resolution Authorizing a Study of the Problems of the Aged and Aging. pp. 43 and 64. US Govn. Printing Office, Washington, DC, 1988.

7. Ibid.35.

8. Ibid. 37.

9. Fact Sheet on Spousal Improverishment—Files of Bluegrass LTC Ombudsman.

10. Ibid. 39.

11. Ibid. 40.

12. Op. cit., Linkletter, 142-44.

13. Film: "What Do You See, Nurse?" (Files Bluegrass LTC Ombudsman, Lexington, Ky.)

14. Kentucky Association of Mental Health.

Chapter 18

1 *Better Homes and Gardens* Magazine, November 1988, Meredith Corp., Des Moines, IA 50386, 51-60.

2. *Development in Aging: 1987*, Vol. 3, "The Long-Term Care", Special Committee on Aging, US Senate, 22.

3. *Parent Care*, Jan/Feb. 1990, "Games Patients Play" 6.

4. Pamplet from Cabinet for Human Resources, Frankfort, Ky. Warning Signs. Reprinted with permission from *Modern Maturity*, Copyright 1987, AARP.

5. *Parent Care*, Sept/Oct 1989, "Resources to Assist Family Caregivers." Univ. of Kansas, Gerontology Center, Vol. 4, #6.

General—"Aging parents: Coping with the Stress Caused by a Parent's Dependency" by Rita H. Smart, Madison County Extension Agent, Home Economics, Kentucky, April 1989, *Blue Grass RECC*

Chapter 20

1. *Developments in Aging: 1987*, Vol.3, The Long-Term Care Challenge, A Report of the Special Committee on Aging, US Senate, Jan. 28, 1987, 46-47.
2. James Halpern, Ph. D., *Helping Your Aging Parents*, Ballentine Books, 1987, 148.
3. Ibid: 161
4. Marjory M. Blood, *Characteristics of Care: Hospice Versus Nursing Home*, Paper given at the 7th Annual Meeting, National Citizens Coalition for Nursing Home Reform, May 18, 1983.
5. Ibid. 224.
6. Ibid. 225-26.
7. Art Linkletter, *Old Age Is Not For Sissies* (Penguin Books, 1989), 130-32

Conclusion

1. "Touching Shoulders," *Masterpieces of Religious Verse*, James Dalton Morrison, ed. (Harper and Row, 1948), 390.